Psionic Medicine

Psionic Medicine

The study and treatment of the causative factors in illness

J. H. Reyner BSC, DIC, FIEE
in collaboration with
George Laurence MRCS, LRCP, FRCS (Edin)
and
Carl Upton LDS (Birm)

SAMUEL WEISER, INC.,
NEW YORK, N.Y. 10003

First published in 1974
by Routledge & Kegan Paul Ltd, London
First published in the United States of America, 1974
by Samuel Weiser, Inc.
New York, N.Y. 10003

Set in 11 on 12 Imprint
and printed in Great Britain by
T. & A. Constable Ltd, Edinburgh

ISBN 0-87728-272-2

Contents

Foreword by George Laurence MRCS, LRCP, FRCS (Edin) vii

1 A New Dimension in Medicine 1

2 The Unmanifest Reality 11

3 Etheric Body 17

4 Homoeopathy 24

5 Miasms and Toxins 30

6 The Unitary Theory of Disease 40

7 Extra-sensory Perception 47

8 The Dowser's Pendulum 55

9 Medical Dowsing 61

10 The Basis of Psionic Medical Technique 67

11 Causative Factors in Illness 73

12 The Psionic Method in Dental Medicine 79

13 Psionic Medicine in Practice 85

14 The Whole Man 92

Appendices

1 Simple Exercises with a Pendulum preparatory to Medical Dowsing 97

2 Commentary by George Laurence on McDonagh's Unitary Concept of Disease 106

3 Clinical Cases 111

4 The Formative Forces in Cancer 132

Further Reading 135

Index 137

Illustrations

Figure 1	Illustrating how a surface, having two dimensions, contains infinite possibilities for the world of lines	19
Figure 2	Illustrating a shadow created in the world of the surface dwellers by an object existing in a superior world	22
Figure 3	The Dowser's Pendulum	98
Figure 4	The Laurence Chart used in medical dowsing	104

Foreword

by George Laurence MRCS, LRCP, FRCS (Edin)

I find it most gratifying that a scientist of Mr Reyner's standing should be so deeply convinced of the value of psionic methods of diagnosis.

As a doctor for over sixty-five years, I am disappointed with the lack of progress in medicine, especially as compared with that in surgery and other allied fields. Every day countless treatments and cures are advertised, but the majority of these are based on new synthetic chemicals—and causation has been ignored. The psionic principle looks for the cause of deviation from normal health before trying to deal with symptoms.

It is my hope that the book will stimulate interest in this important branch of medical science.

Chapter 1

A New Dimension in Medicine

There are epochs in medical history when the trend of knowledge is significantly changed. One can cite Harvey's classical treatise on the circulation of the blood in 1628, or the work of Louis Pasteur in 1865 which led to the now accepted antiseptic techniques. Yet another landmark was the discovery of penicillin by Fleming in 1938 which ushered in the era of antibiotics and the widespread chemotherapy of today.

Concurrently there has been a vast expansion of knowledge of the physical structure of living matter, both in respect of the intricate structure of the cells and in the communication between them, as a result of which medical practice has been able to devise new treatments for many bodily ailments, often with spectacular success. These very successes, however, have tended to create an undue reliance on the material aspects of medicine, in the belief that a full understanding of the physical mechanisms will ultimately provide a cure for all the ailments of the flesh.

This is an illusion, for although an intelligent application of material knowledge can often produce an amelioration of the conditions, the clinical symptoms are really only the physical evidence of some disturbance of the vital energy of the body. This is not, in itself, a new philosophy, having been held, if not always acknowledged, for at least 2500 years. In fact Hippocrates, revered as the Father of Medicine, is reported to have said that disease does not appear purely as a malady (*pathos*) but is significantly accompanied by an exertion (*ponos*) by the body itself to restore the disturbed equilibrium of its functions. This inherent healing power is known as the *Vis Medicatrix Naturae*, and the enlightened physician is well aware that his true role is to assist the operations of an intelligence which is considerably greater than his own, as has been pointed out with a characteristic sense of wonder by Sir Charles Sherrington in his classic book *Man on his Nature*.

The problem, of course, lies in communicating with this intelligence, because it does not use the language of the material senses, but there have been certain developments in recent years which make it possible to communicate, scientifically and practically, with the vital energies in the body. This requires the use of the extrasensory faculties which used to be regarded as haphazard, but of which the existence is now scientifically accepted. There is an established science of parapsychology which is concerned with the investigation of these inherent, but normally dormant, *psi* functions, as they are called; and their application to medical practice is therefore known as psionic medicine.

We shall see that this permits a much wider understanding of the human organism, of which the physical body is only a part, thereby introducing a new dimension into the applications of orthodox techniques. This constitutes a significant advance in medical knowledge, which many well-qualified and experienced practitioners believe heralds the advent of a new epoch in the treatment of disease.

Scientific discoveries are often ahead of their time and do not gain acceptance until developments in other directions have produced the right climate. In this sense, psionic medicine can be regarded as originating from the work of Samuel Hahnemann, whose *Organon der rationelle Heilkunde*, published in 1810, sought to rationalize the ancient but hitherto haphazard art of homoeopathy.

This is the technique of administering, in minute doses, medicaments which in a healthy person actually produce the disease under treatment; but this is an over-simplification because although Hahnemann's initial researches were based on this principle of 'like is cured by like', he subsequently found that the efficacy of the remedies was increased by a specific form of dilution called potentizing (which we shall discuss later), which virtually eliminated any physical trace of the original substance.

This led him to believe that the curative properties were not derived from the chemical properties of the substances, but from some subtle form of energy which they possessed, which was in some way preserved by his process of potentizing; and he contended that the proper administration of these remedies reinforced certain vital energies inherent in the organism. He says specifically in his *Organon*:

> In the healthy condition of man the spiritual vital force, the dynamis that animates the material body . . . maintains all parts of the organism in harmonious operation. When a person falls ill it is because this vital force, everywhere present in his organism, has become deranged by the influence of some morbific agent inimical to life.

These ideas received very limited acceptance in the material climate of his time, the more so since the subtle energies which he postulated cannot be understood in terms of the ordinary senses. To communicate with them a certain quality of intuition is required, which is customarily regarded with suspicion.

Today, it is accepted that the information provided by the physical senses is of a severely restricted character, and that the familiar world is only a limited portrayal of a much larger realm which is not manifest to the senses. We shall discuss this more fully later, but it will suffice to note here that we are equipped with a range of paranormal senses which can respond to the influences of this superior world, in which exist the real causes and relationships of physical appearances.

The real significance of Hahnemann's philosophy was its dependence on this paranormal sensitivity. He believed that the correct approach was to treat the patient and not the disease. There are, of course, many orthodox practitioners who have a similarly enlightened approach but the vast availability of modern specifics, and their apparently much more rapid effectiveness, inevitably tends to strengthen the reliance on physical medicaments.

Hahnemann painstakingly prepared a *Materia Medica* of some hundred preparations which had been proved by experiment to contain the appropriate corrective energies for a wide range of ailments. Today the list has been developed to include some 2000 items, but these are not regarded as specifics so much as guides to assist the practitioner to determine the real causes of the malady. There is a certain element of exploration—as with orthodox practice—but it is directed to the discovery of the true nature of the disturbances (which Hahnemann called miasms) responsible for the symptoms; and the efficacy of the diagnosis and subsequent treatment is clearly dependent to a considerable extent on the intuition of the practitioner.

It was natural, therefore, that efforts should be made to assess these paranormal influences more objectively. This was not possible in Hahnemann's time, but towards the end of the nineteenth century the discovery of X-rays and other 'invisible' radiations prompted several doctors to wonder whether the concept of vital energy might not, after all, be valid. Among these was the distinguished American physician Albert Abrams who had studied in Europe under such famous masters as Virchow, Wassermann and von Helmholtz. He conceived the idea that all matter might possess its own intrinsic radiation—an idea somewhat ahead of its time, though one finds a hint of it in the writings of the seventeenth-century mystic Jacob Boehme, who speaks of 'the signature of all things'. Hence Abrams argued that if a suitable detecting instrument could be devised it should be possible to tune in to the radiations of different organs of the body, and so arrive at a scientific basis of diagnosis.

The problem was how to detect such radiation. It did not appear to be electromagnetic in character—and in fact is not—so that no orthodox equipment was suitable. However, during a routine examination of a patient suffering from cancer (of the lip) he observed a dull note when percussing a certain area of the abdomen. He subsequently found that he obtained a similar reaction on a healthy young man in close contact with a cancer specimen—or even connected thereto by a wire—from which he deduced that some subtle energy was being radiated by the unhealthy tissue.

He endeavoured to quantify the effect by introducing a resistance box into the 'circuit' and found that at a certain setting the reaction disappeared; and he then found that if he used other diseased tissues as a reference he obtained similar reactions, but at different resistance settings. Still later he discovered that the reactions could be obtained by replacing the actual patient with a sample in the form of a blood spot, or sample of hair or urine. This led to the development of the celebrated Abrams Box, by which a patient's sample could be analysed by reference to an empirically-determined register of vibration rates relevant to specific ailments.

The method attracted the attention of other investigators,

notably Ruth Drown in America and George de la Warr in England, who devised their own forms of instrument, and considerable interest began to develop in this technique of radiesthesia, as it was called. Its efficacy depended upon a combination of intuitive sensitivity and sound medical knowledge, and under these conditions encouraging results were obtained. Unfortunately the instruments were leased or sold to all and sundry without respect for qualifications, as a result of which many grossly unscientific, and even stupid, interpretations were made, which brought the system into grave disrepute.

Partly for this reason, and partly from prejudice, it was spurned by the orthodox profession who found it difficult to understand the possibility of diagnosis and treatment without the physical presence of the patient. Nevertheless, in 1924 a committee was appointed by the British Medical Association, under the chairmanship of Sir Thomas (later Lord) Horder, which somewhat unexpectedly reported that the diagnostic possibilities of the system appeared to have some validity; but since this was not accompanied by any recommendation for further research no official move was made to pursue the matter.

Radiesthesia, however, had received an impetus from another quarter. It had long been known that certain individuals possessed the ability to locate the presence of subterranean water, or deposits of metallic ores, by holding in their hands a forked hazel twig which exhibited a pronounced and uncontrollable movement when passing over the hidden substance. The effect was believed to be produced by an extra-sensory rapport between the mind of the operator and the object of the search, which produced involuntary muscular movements.

The art became known as dowsing, from an old Cornish word meaning to strike, and has been found to have many applications other than water-divining. Moreover, other forms of detector can be used, and for many purposes a small pendulum is more convenient. We shall discuss it in detail later, for it is a genuine art of considerable value in the development of the paranormal senses. It was extensively developed during the early years of the present century by the Abbé Mermet, a French priest who acquired considerable expertise with the pendulum, and whose standard work on the subject *Principles and Practice of Radiesthesia* contains records of many remarkable achievements over a period of some forty years. A significant aspect of his work was the development of quantitative techniques which began to raise the process from an art to a science.

In the medical field a similar quest was pursued by a number of eminent doctors, in the forefront of whom was Guyon Richards, and later George Laurence; and it was the latter who was subsequently to make a significant advance in medical practice by integrating the techniques of radiesthesia and homoeopathy into a practical unity. Laurence was a surgeon of distinction who had become increasingly dissatisfied with the orthodox preoccupation with symptoms. In his own words, he says:

> I had a growing conviction that I did not always know what I was really doing—or rather why I was doing it. In other words, I did not know *why* people were ill.
>
> It was fairly easy to treat ordinary infectious diseases and acute ailments, but when it came to chronic disorders such as malignant diseases, rheumatism, degenerate nervous troubles, and other so-called incurable maladies, we did not know the 'why', and were reduced to treating names and labels, signs and symptoms, without a clue as to causation; and hence the temporary alleviation of symptoms was the best that I, or any of my contemporaries, could do.

By one of life's chances (which the philosophers say are not as accidental as they may appear) he came into contact with Dr Guyon Richards and was introduced to the idea of medical dowsing. This proved to be the key for which he had been seeking, for he had long been convinced that the physical body is only part of a much larger structure which is not recognizable by the ordinary senses. He believed that it was within this unmanifest realm that the vital energies operated, and he found that by the use of the pendulum he was able to detect the derangements of these energies responsible for the physical and psychological disturbances which produced the clinical symptoms.

He then found that by an extension of the technique he was able to determine appropriate treatment which would restore the vital harmony—usually, but not necessarily, by homoeopathic medicaments—and so for the first time was able to formulate a scientific method of diagnosing and treating the basic causes of illness. This he developed with patience and assiduity over the years, and has now established a technique which he and his colleagues have applied for over a quarter of a century with remarkable success, often disclosing the hidden causes and appropriate treatment of many chronic and supposedly incurable diseases, as is exemplified in some of the case histories quoted later.

The system depends essentially on the exercise of the paranormal senses, of which the existence is now scientifically accepted; and because by convention the Greek letter *psi* has been adopted in this connotation, Laurence calls his system psionic medicine, of which the various aspects will be considered in detail in the chapters which follow.

The significant feature of psionic medicine is that it is not just another fringe technique but is a means of extending existing orthodox knowledge from the part to the whole. Nor is it merely an offshoot of radiesthesia, for the extra-sensory faculty is not used as an end in itself, but as part of an integrated system which involves a knowledge of homoeopathy allied to a thorough and practical experience of orthodox medical principles.

George Laurence knew from a very early age that he wanted to be a doctor, and in due course enrolled as a medical student at Liverpool University, where the Professor of Physics was Oliver Lodge (later Sir Oliver), whose ideas on the then new concepts of ether waves made an early impact. He subsequently went to St George's Hospital, London, where he qualified in 1904, following which he occupied himself with increasing distinction in a variety of hospital appointments and private practice.

In 1915 he gained the Fellowship in Surgery at Edinburgh, and later that year bought a third share in a practice in Chippenham, Wiltshire. Almost immediately his two senior partners were called up for war service, and he was left to carry on the practice alone, which involved a number of local hospital and consultative appointments which continued for nearly forty years.

During this period he had become increasingly concerned with causation and had begun to develop his concept of psionic analysis; and in 1954 he retired to Wargrave in Berkshire to devote himself exclusively to the practice of psionic medicine. His activities attracted the attention of other qualified practitioners, and in 1968 a group of doctors and dental surgeons formed the Psionic Medical Society to promote the wider practical application of the system, with Dr George Laurence, MRCS, LRCP, FRCS (Edin) as President. The Vice-President is Dr Aubrey Westlake BA, MB, BChir, MRCS, LRCP, whose writings and lectures on medical dowsing are well known, while the Secretary is Carl Upton LDS (Birm).

Born into an English farming family, Carl Upton entered the Medical Faculty of Birmingham University where he studied dentistry in the Dental School of the Faculty. Throughout his training the emphasis was on the need for close collaboration with medical colleagues at all times, which materially influenced his outlook. After qualifying he spent two years in private practice before entering the Army Medical Service, in which he served for eight years at home and in the Middle East. He was then posted to the War Office as Deputy Assistant Director, Army Dental Service, which occupied him during the second half of the war.

At the close of the war he was sent for training in maxillo-facial dental surgery at the Victoria Hospital, East Grinstead, under Sir Archibald McIndoe, and was subsequently appointed Command Specialist Dental Surgeon to a home command, and later to India and Singapore. In 1948 he retired from the Army and entered private practice in South Africa, where he stayed for some years, working in close collaboration with his medical colleagues in local hospitals.

During this period he developed an increasing interest in the preventive aspects of dentistry, and took every opportunity to investigate any ideas, whether orthodox or not, which could throw light on the basic causes of dental disorders, in the pursuit of which he was greatly assisted by his wide travels and meetings with people of many races and types. On his return to England in 1963 he increasingly devoted his attention to the possibilities of homoeopathy in relation to dental conditions; and having come into contact with Westlake, and later Laurence, he realized that the fulfilment of his quest lay in the integrated philosophy of psionic medicine.

He therefore put himself in the hands of Laurence to receive a thorough training in the techniques, and in 1968 retired from active dental surgical practice to devote his attention to the furtherance of the reconciliation between medical science and the traditional healing arts to which psionic medicine holds an important key.

The conferences and journals of the Psionic Medical Society are attracting increasing interest among medical practitioners who feel with Laurence (and Hahnemann before him) the need to treat the patient rather than the disease. It is felt that the time is now ripe for an authoritative treatise on the subject, which I have been asked to write. I have agreed to do this with some humility, for my background is scientific rather than medical. Yet my philosophical researches have convinced me that the world of the senses is a very limited portrayal of a much greater reality, so that the application of this concept to medical practice appears to me to be fundamentally sound. This I hope to establish in the chapters which follow, with the collaboration of George Laurence and Carl Upton in the medical aspects.

We have given considerable attention to the format, for the object is not to create a widespread popular appeal, which would only embarrass the limited facilities at present available. Nor is it desirable to provide detailed medical information on the application of the techniques, because this might encourage the indiscriminate use of the methods by insufficiently qualified operators; and we have already seen the damage which this caused in the early development of radiesthesia so that today the term is regarded by many people with opprobrium. Psionic medicine is based on a very precise application of the paranormal faculties, which can only be effectively employed after strict and controlled training.

The book is therefore directed to those members of the orthodox medical profession who are beginning to mistrust the present preoccupation with the amelioration of clinical symptoms, and who are prepared to believe that these are only the manifestation of deeper underlying causes, to the discovery of which their skills could be more profitably employed. As we have seen, this requires a radical reorientation of thought, based on the understanding that the interpretations of the ordinary senses can only provide a very limited portrayal of reality.

The first part of the book will thus be concerned with a scientific assessment of the existence and characteristics of the unmanifest realms which contain the real causes and relationships of physical behaviour, and the possibilities of identifying these underlying patterns. We shall then consider the methods devised by Laurence for the practical interpretation of the ideas, illustrated by selected case histories. It will be seen that the techniques do not supersede but reinforce orthodox knowledge, which is an essential prerequisite. One is reminded of the early days of electronics, which acquired a certain mystique, resulting in unnecessary and even incorrect applications in preference to straightforward methods. Similarly, orthodox medicine is adequate and right for many purposes, but is unable to cope with certain recalcitrant disorders, for which a more subtle form of therapy is required. This is the role of psionic medicine.

Chapter 2

The Unmanifest Reality

From the brief introduction in the preceding chapter it will be seen that psionic medicine is basically concerned with the intangible energies which maintain the bodily functions. It regards all disease as resulting from derangements of this vital energy, which produce the clinical symptoms recognized by the ordinary senses; and it seeks to cure these physical aberrations by restoring the vital harmony.

This is indeed a fundamental tenet of true medicine, but in the present material age it is apt to be regarded as an abstract idea. There is, however, nothing abstract about psionic techniques, which are entirely practical; but the energies with which they are concerned are not of a physical character but operate within a superior realm which is not manifest to the ordinary senses, and it is essential to recognize the existence of this unmanifest world, not as a mere theory but as an actual reality.

Hence before discussing the techniques in detail we must consider briefly the structure of the unmanifest world. This does not involve abstruse metaphysics but simply a willingness to think beyond the limitations of conventional acceptance. We shall see that the appearance and behaviour of the familiar environment is an interpretation by a very restricted range of senses of a pattern of an entirely superior order; and more significantly, that all ordinary knowledge is subject to similar limitations.

There is in most of us an innate awareness of the existence of a superior world, though usually as a matter of religious belief rather than practical conviction. Yet the existence of an immaterial world is now accepted by scientific opinion, which can no longer formulate adequate concepts in purely material terms, and is therefore seeking to reconcile physical knowledge with what Arthur Koestler has called man's intuitive intimations of deeper levels of reality.

Let us then examine some of the processes which we normally take for granted. How are we aware of the world in which we live? How, indeed, do we know that we exist? The knowledge is derived in the first place from the evidence of the five physical senses. These are extremely elegant mechanisms of response to stimulus—which incidentally are not confined to man—which receive impressions from the environment and feed this information, in the form of electrical signals, to a remarkably sophisticated computer called the Central Nervous System, located mainly (but not entirely) in the brain. Here they are analysed by reference to a previously established pattern of associations—partly innate, but mainly acquired by experience—as a result of which appropriate action is generated.

The process is so rapid as to be virtually instantaneous, and is so automatic that it is rarely questioned. Yet actually these interpretations are of an extraordinarily limited character, for several reasons, of which the most significant is that the senses which supply the basic information only operate within certain specific limits. For example, the human ear only responds to sounds within a range of approximately 30 to 16,000 vibrations per second (and as one grows older the upper limit becomes progressively and often seriously reduced). Yet animals and birds have different hearing ranges, which partly overlap the human range, but include a response to vibrations of much higher pitch which are inaudible to our ears. This fact is utilized in the 'silent' dog whistles which emit a sound too shrill for the human ear but to which a dog immediately responds. Even higher frequencies are employed by bats in their remarkable radar system which employs short bursts of supersonic waves which are reflected from obstacles in their path; and there are man-made vibrations of still higher frequency used in a variety of modern techniques. Human hearing, in fact, only responds to a fraction of the available range of vibrations in the physical realm.

The sense of sight is even more restricted. The eyes respond to a small range of vibrations of a different character, known as electromagnetic waves, which are reflected in varying degree by the objects of the familiar world. Most objects only reflect some of the waves and thereby exhibit a characteristic colour, but the whole range of colours is contained within what is actually a very small span of vibrations, constituting an almost negligible fraction of the vast spectrum of electric waves known to science. These extend from the alpha rhythms of the brain, through the gamut of radio waves to the infra-red rays which produce the sensation of heat. Then follows the tiny band of vibrations called visible light, followed by ultra-violet rays, X-rays, and gamma rays, culminating in the cosmic rays which reach us from outer space. In all there are over fifty octaves of these electromagnetic radiations, of which visible light occupies rather less than one octave. If our eyes responded to an even slightly different range of vibrations—for example, X-rays—the whole appearance of the world, and its occupants, would be entirely different. In place of the familiar surroundings (which would become invisible) there would be a completely altered environment.

All the senses, in fact, only respond to a strictly limited range of impressions sufficient to maintain a satisfactory relationship to the environment. Anything more would impose an unnecessary overload on the brain, which could be disastrous; and this prompted the Cambridge philosopher C. D. Broad to suggest that the function of the brain was to act as a reducing valve. Whether one regards this as resulting from intelligent design or the process of evolution is immaterial. (The two are not incompatible anyway.) The significant point is that all ordinary awareness, and behaviour, is based on associations which have been derived primarily from very limited perceptions.

The range of perception has been enormously extended by many ingenious artefacts. The realm of the very large can be probed by telescopes, using both optical and radio methods, while at the other end of the scale are the microscopes, including electron types which permit one to 'see' atoms. Yet the wealth of conjectural knowledge derived from these explorations is still based on the intelligent interpretation of information primarily supplied by the physical senses, and is thereby inherently limited.

In the light of these observations one can understand why Hindu philosophy says that we live in a world of illusion (*maya*). This does not mean that life is a figment of the imagination, for it clearly has a very real existence in practical terms. The word illusion comes from a Latin root meaning to play a game, so that one can envisage the appearances and happenings of the familiar world as the portrayal, in accordance with certain specific but restricted rules, of the conditions existing in a much more comprehensive real world.

Plato likened the situation to that of a cave-dweller who sees the world outside only through a narrow slit which slowly moves to disclose further portions of the landscape. It is an apt analogy, for it is characteristic of the physical senses that they only respond to impressions in sequence, so that the moving slit can be regarded as representing a transit of consciousness through the real world which creates the illusion of passing time. The cave-dweller is aware of a succession of impressions which will constitute his life. To a small extent there may be a connection between one incident and the next, but the overall sequence will appear quite arbitrary. Moreover because of his limited vision the events of yesterday will appear irrevocably past and those of tomorrow not yet created; whereas in fact he is merely obtaining successive glimpses of an already-existing landscape.

By inference we can postulate that the whole of the phenomenal world—the pattern of objects and events displayed by the senses—is created by the transit of a certain level of consciousness through an already-existing domain of a superior order. This real world can be regarded as a fabric of virtually infinite possibilities, some of which are actualized by the moving finger of time. So that the past has not gone for ever, and the future is already waiting (though not rigidly predestined since consciousness has certain degrees of freedom as we shall see later).

This is an idea which can provide a new background to one's awareness. Not so long ago it would have been dismissed as abstract speculation, of interest only to philosophers and mystics. But scientific thought is increasingly accepting the existence of realms beyond the perceptions of the physical senses. For example, an Australian astronomer, Dr Vidal of Mount Stromlo Observatory, recently announced the discovery of two 'black holes' in the universe relatively close at hand (in astronomical terms). A black hole is a region in space where the remains of a once-giant star appear to have vanished altogether out of the universe! This poses a problem of the first magnitude, for how can matter cease to exist?

The theory is that while it ceases to exist in that region of space, it moves into another universe, which Professor John A. Wheeler of Princeton, one of the world's most distinguished physicists, calls Superspace—a universe that lasts for ever, while others come and go. According to this theory, the matter of all the galaxies came originally from Superspace, into which it will ultimately return, to be replaced by a new universe (not necessarily obeying the same laws as the present one).

This is an idea which contains a substratum of truth; yet it is couched in terms which involve the curious reluctance of physicists to admit the existence of a Higher Intelligence which can be neither perceived nor apprehended by the ordinary senses. Such is the conditioning of the habitual sense-based associations that we tend to envisage superior realms in terms of some kind of super-materiality. Admittedly, since Einstein's classic formulation $e=mc^2$, we regard matter and energy as interchangeable, but we are still thinking in physical terms.

It is necessary to transcend these limited interpretations and envisage a real world of a different quality which can only be comprehended by the deeper levels of the mind, which are intuitive. In these terms the unmanifest realm must be envisaged as a kind of force-field in which the interplay of cosmic consciousness creates manifestations at the phenomenal level which appear as matter or energy. Such a concept has many implications which can provide an understanding of normally inexplicable phenomena.

We shall see, for example, that the matter/energies of the sense-based world are only a part of the manifestations of the real world; and that there are other forms of energy which do not fall within the conventional pattern, but which can be detected by the paranormal senses. There is, indeed, scientific evidence which suggests that matter is being continuously created out of the eternal fabric of the unmanifest force-field. Clearly, the belief that the world of the senses is the only reality is ludicrously naïve.

In practical terms, we are concerned only with those manifestations which fall within the ambit of human intelligence and consciousness; but in the ordinary way the available possibilities are only utilized to a very limited extent. For example, it is popularly supposed that increasing detail implies increased consciousness, whereas they are really in inverse ratio. As a small-scale example, consider the production of an aircraft. The mind of the designer will envisage a comprehensive range of possibilities, including an understanding of the laws of flight. From this will emerge a succession of increasingly particularized specifications culminating in a mass of detailed drawings and schedules. Each stage involves an appropriate intelligence, of a high quality at its level, but of progressively decreasing order relative to that of the original designer. Hence the increasing preoccupation with material knowledge today is actually an exercise of a decreasing order of consciousness, leading ever farther from the truth.

Consciousness means, literally, knowing all together, and it is quite obvious that our ordinary awareness falls far short of this. One has only to consider the world of organic life, which we take for granted. This is controlled by a stupendous intelligence which organizes the response of plants to the succeeding seasons, the habits and behaviour of birds and animals, the interrelated functioning of insects and micro-organisms, all in an ordered and co-ordinated pattern. The botanist or biologist may have a detailed knowledge of the mechanisms involved, but this in no way constitutes a full awareness. Organic life, in fact, is directed by a consciousness of an entirely incommensurable order.

Still less are we aware of our body, which again we take for granted. Yet it is a wonderfully co-ordinated structure of millions of cells, of variously specialized types, each of which performs its appropriate function subject to the overall direction of a controlling intelligence. Medical science provides detailed knowledge of the mechanisms, but this does not, *per se*, constitute awareness.

Our so-called consciousness, in fact, is normally occupied with the limited awareness of personal desires which in the scale of the Universe are utterly trivial. So that to attain any true understanding we have to awaken from our habitual lethargy and stretch our minds to embrace wider horizons.

As mentioned earlier, this is not an exercise of abstract metaphysics. It involves the practical recognition of the fact that all phenomenal appearance and behaviour is a portrayal by a very limited range of senses of a much greater but unmanifest reality; and therefore all ordinary knowledge and reasoning, which is derived from these same senses, is subject to the same limitations. This is a most important proviso. It does not mean that ordinary knowledge is to be decried; on the contrary it is of great value, at its level, and should awaken a profound feeling of wonder. But to regard it as total precludes any possibility of real understanding.

Chapter 3

Etheric Body

It is not difficult to accept the idea that the familiar world interpreted by the ordinary senses is only a very limited portrayal of reality. Yet with a curious blindness this is not deemed to apply to our own body, with which we normally identify ourselves completely. A more intelligent and practical understanding is achieved by the recognition that the physical body is merely a part of a larger entity existing in the unmanifest world.

Esoteric philosophy regards the material body as a temporary habitation for a spiritual body of much greater potentialities, which is itself a structure of levels animated by successively higher consciousness. In practical terms, however, it is sufficient to recognize that the physical body, with its wonderfully contrived patterns of behaviour, is only an interpretation by the senses of a structure of a superior order of intelligence in the real world.

This real structure constitutes what is known as the etheric body. The term is sometimes regarded askance, as a theosophical abstraction redolent of the nineteenth-century belief in a universal non-physical medium called the ether, which is now outmoded. Yet scientific opinion is beginning to accept that the concept may have a certain validity in the interpretation of a now-acknowledged superior world beyond the evidence of the senses, so that the idea of an etheric world need no longer be regarded as unscientific.

It is a characteristic of the physical world, which is usually taken completely for granted, that it permits communication at a distance. The sounds to which our ears respond are produced by events taking place some distance away, maybe only a few feet but sometimes several miles. Even more remarkably, we see the world around us as a result of an intangible communication between our eyes and a variety of objects mostly beyond the range of physical contact, even billions of miles away in the case of the stars in the heavens. We explain this by saying that the intelligence is communicated by vibrations, which are rhythmic changes of condition to which the senses (or other detecting devices) respond. But any such disturbances necessarily involve the existence of some medium through which they can be transmitted.

Sounds are transmitted by a physical jostling between the molecules of the air, as is demonstrated by the well-known classroom experiment of enclosing an electric bell within a glass jar connected to a vacuum pump. As the air is extracted by the pump the sound gradually ceases although the bell can be seen to be still operating. But the vibrations which produce the effects of visible light (and the many other phenomena mentioned in the previous chapter) do not take place within any physical medium, for they travel equally well in a vacuum, or through outer space; and exhaustive experiments towards the end of the last century utterly failed to disclose the existence of any tangible medium in which they could operate.

Science therefore postulated the existence of some all-pervading, non-physical medium called the ether, through which these vibrations could travel; but the idea was abhorrent to the material mind and it was discarded in favour of the mathematical concept of the space-time continuum, which was more acceptable to logical reasoning. Yet this is really only a change of approach, and there is today an increasing acknowledgment of the existence of superior realms beyond the evidence of the senses.

From what has already been said it will be clear that the search for abstruse mathematical explanations is self-defeating, since the true conditions cannot be interpreted in these terms. A more real, and practical, understanding can be obtained from the concept of the etheric realm, which can be regarded as a fabric within the real world in which the interplay of influences at that level creates the manifestations which appear in the phenomenal world as vibrations. Many of these take the form of the familiar radiations of physical science, but we shall see that there are other forms of manifestation to which the ordinary senses do not respond, but which can be detected by the little-used paranormal senses.

We can only assess the nature of the etheric world by inference. Yet scientific progress in general is based on intelligent conjecture, for which one then seeks verification. We accept the existence of atoms and electrons, though we cannot see them, because they appear to provide an understanding of observed effects. We can make similar conjectures about the equally unmanifest etheric world, with the proviso that it will, by definition, be subject to laws of a superior order which will transcend the limitations of the phenomenal world.

Its most significant feature is that, like the landscape in Plato's analogy, which the cave-dweller only sees piecemeal, it has a continuing existence. So we can envisage that it is some kind of transit through this (for us) eternal pattern which produces the

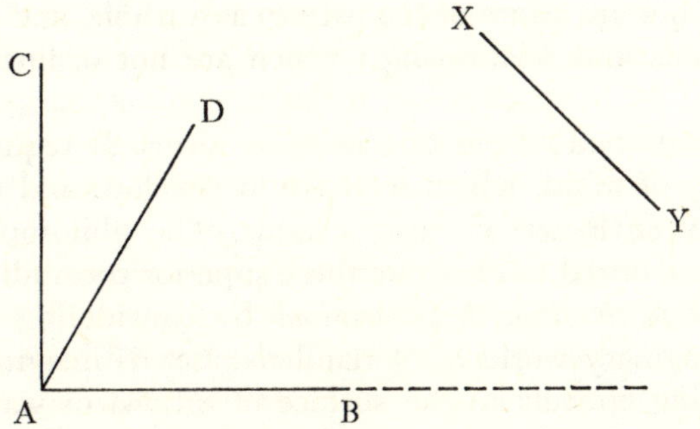

Figure 1 *Illustrating how a surface, having two dimensions, contains infinite possibilities for the world of lines*

manifestations in the phenomenal world. These provide impressions which the ordinary senses interpret in succession, thereby creating the illusions of time and space; but the etheric realm is not subject to these limitations so that any event or situation may have its origin in a part of the eternal fabric which exists, for us, in another part of time.

The etheric world, in fact, contains an additional dimension. This is nothing mysterious but simply means that it possesses an extra degree of freedom. We can illustrate this quite simply by the diagram in Figure 1. The line AB is produced by the movement of a point from A to B. Any further movement in this direction can only produce a longer line, i.e. an extension of its length. But the surface of the paper contains the possibility of movement in a variety of other directions such as AC or AD. Lines can be drawn which start from some entirely different place, such as XY; and other lines can be drawn which go back on their tracks, creating circles or spirals. All this is possible because the surface contains an additional degree of freedom which permits movement in a different dimension, so that the surface contains the possibility of an infinite number of lines.

Similarly the etheric world is a realm which contains for us infinite possibilities. The course of events results from the actualization of a specific part of the pattern but it is entirely possible for other 'lines' to be created, or for an existing sequence to be modified. We shall see later that we possess a range of paranormal senses which do not respond to impressions in isolated sequence, but are aware of the pattern as a whole, and can thus see connections and relationships which are not ordinarily apparent.

We are not accustomed to thinking in these terms. It requires a certain flexibility of mind, which we have to develop; and this can be assisted by analogies of various kinds. The philosopher C. H. Hinton endeavoured to illustrate these superior possibilities in his book *What is the Fourth Dimension?* by considering the situation of an imaginary world of 'flatlanders'. Let us imagine a race of beings living entirely in the surface of a bowl of water. They would be aware of only two dimensions—length and breadth—but would have no appreciation of height. If we insert some object—say one's finger—into the bowl, it will create in the surface of the liquid a roughly circular obstruction which will enter the surface world mysteriously and without any apparent cause or reason. It will move around and even change its shape in a quite arbitrary manner. It may destroy numbers of the surface dwellers in what to them would be an inexplicable catastrophe. Yet to us, with our awareness of the additional dimension of height, there is no mystery. The finger was inserted for some simple purpose, and any disturbance of the surface of the liquid is purely incidental.

It is a simple matter to extend this analogy to our own situation. We live in a three-dimensional world which we have seen to be a cross-section of a more real world having an entirely superior degree of freedom—which the mathematician would call a fourth dimension. So the familiar succession of events is a pattern which is not derived solely from the operation of logical cause and effect, but is influenced by the interplay of forces in the real world, which can produce apparently arbitrary and even inexplicable results in the phenomenal world, but which are quite normal and meaningful at the superior level.

It is in this real world that the etheric body exists, as a pattern which is progressively scanned by the moving finger of time. This creates the physical body, of which we are normally only aware of the present condition; but this is actually continually changing in time from birth to death, so that even in material terms the day-to-day appearance is only a fraction of the whole. Yet this is only a shadow of the real entity, for the developing conditions of the physical body are all created by successive interpretations by the senses of an underlying structure in the real world.

Thus the etheric body can be seen as an established, and already-existing, pattern within the timeless fabric of relatively infinite possibilities. It is not unalterable and can be modified to a minor extent, though the basic pattern can only be varied by a change in the spiritual quality of the individual, with which we are not concerned here. It will be clear, however, that the events of life, and specifically the bodily functions, are subject to two kinds of influence. There are first the ordinary laws of cause and effect which apply to the phenomenal world in general; but there are also effects arising from unmanifest causes in the etheric body, which are much more subtle, and can result from deviations in any part of the etheric pattern, in which the relationships entirely transcend the limitations of space and time.

To think in these terms makes it possible to appreciate an entirely superior order of relationships. Every object and event in the phenomenal world has its counterpart in the etheric realm in which there are subtle and usually unsuspected connections. The physical body is an interpretation by the senses of the etheric body, which is a specific pattern in the unmanifest realm; and this pattern is connected with the corresponding patterns of other people, and objects, not necessarily confined within the life-span of the individual in the time of the senses.

We shall see how this approach opens up new fields of practical endeavour, provided that one can recognize the influence of the superior pattern. We can, for example, extend Hinton's analogy by imagining a situation such as is illustrated in Figure 2, which depicts a shadow cast by some object not actually within the surface. This could puzzle the flatlanders who might try all manner of techniques to remove it, without success; but if they could cultivate an awareness of height they might perceive the real cause of the disturbance, which they would then understand and might be able to modify. In similar manner distortions or crystallizations in the etheric body—which Hahnemann called

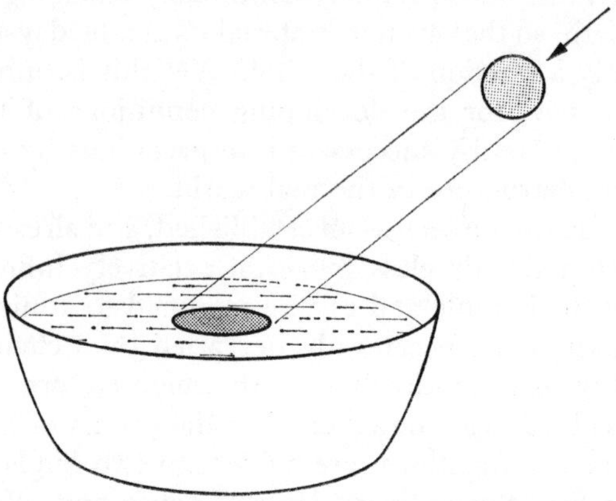

Figure 2 *Illustrating a shadow created in the world of the surface dwellers by an object existing in a superior world*

miasms—can produce shadows in the physical body which manifest themselves as diseases or morbid conditions which will not respond to orthodox treatment.

It is evident that not all ailments have an etheric origin. Some may arise from purely physical contingencies, such as the accidental fracture of a limb or other bodily damage, which can be repaired by orthodox skills; and these skills can be used to ameliorate conditions arising from the natural processes of ageing. But any physical derangement, whether purely mechanical or arising from a toxic infection, impedes the flow of the vital energy; and this the body seeks to restore by its innate intelligence, which resides in the etheric realm. This is the exercise of the *Vis Medicatrix Naturae*, of which the skilled practitioner is intuitively aware, and the recovery can often be assisted by the reinforcement of these vital energies, either by the use of appropriate homoeopathic remedies or simply by the mental acknowledgment of their existence.

The concept of the etheric body thus introduces a new dimension into one's understanding. It reinforces ordinary knowledge by the recognition that the physical body is only part of a much larger unmanifest entity, directed by a superior intelligence. It is with the practical application of this understanding that psionic medicine is concerned.

Chapter 4

Homoeopathy

It is appropriate at this point to consider in more detail the principles of homoeopathy. This has very ancient beginnings, but is usually associated with the name of Samuel Hahnemann who in the early years of the nineteenth century attempted, with some success, to establish the art on a scientific basis. His ideas were not unexpectedly repudiated by the prejudice of his time, and even after one hundred and fifty years have only been partially acknowledged. Nevertheless, the practice is accepted today by the ranks of orthodoxy, partly because it has received a certain royal patronage—both Queen Mary and King George VI were firm believers in its efficacy—but mainly because it is usually regarded as a relatively harmless technique which does not pose any serious threat to established ideas.

Homoeopathy is customarily defined as the treatment of disease by minute doses of drugs which in a healthy person produce symptoms similar to those from which the patient is suffering. This is an interpretation of the ancient adage *similia similibus curentur*—like should be cured by like—found in the Hippocratic writings, as well as in certain early Arabian texts. Actually, this is a gross over-simplification, because the effectiveness of the treatment is not dependent on the drugs as such, but upon certain subtle energies in their constitution which are distilled by a specific method of preparation known as potentizing. The treatment, in fact, is fundamentally dependent on this energy content, which is an entirely different basis of medication, by no means fully appreciated by orthodoxy.

Indeed, Hahnemann himself only came to this realization gradually. He was so disturbed by the brutality of the orthodox medicine of his time that he began to look for gentler remedies; in the course of which he discovered that Peruvian bark (quinine), a recognized specific against ague (but of which he disapproved), could actually induce an appearance of the disease in himself. From this he was led to investigate the effect of small doses of other drugs to find whether they could induce, in a healthy person, symptoms similar to those of specific ailments. For this purpose he enlisted the co-operation of a large number of volunteers among his colleagues and pupils, eschewing tests on animals which he (rightly) believed might not provide valid evidence; and he began to assemble a list of medicaments which he found effective in a variety of superficially unrelated conditions.

For example, a bee sting can produce a distressing and painful oedema, which usually subsides of its own accord; but similar symptoms can result from a variety of internally-generated ailments, and these he found could be cured by minute doses of apis, or bee virus. So he gradually compiled a *Materia Medica* containing over one hundred proven remedies, which has today been enlarged to include some 2000 items.

However, this is only the beginning of the story. Being of a cautious disposition he only administered his remedies in very diluted form, which was fortunate since conventional dosages might have had disastrous results. But he then found, somewhat surprisingly, that increasing the dilution did not reduce the effectiveness, but even in some cases increased it. In an attempt to quantify the process scientifically he introduced, by a stroke of genius, a method of dilution known as potentizing which was to have a profound effect on the results.

In this process the dilution is achieved in a succession of stages, which are known as potencies. For many purposes a decimal dilution is employed. A small, but measured amount of the medicament, usually a simple chemical or herbal substance, is intimately mixed with nine parts of a suitable inert substance. The mixture is violently agitated for a certain length of time, not only to ensure uniform blending but also to produce a certain dissociation of the molecules. One part of this mixture, which is called a 1x potency, is then mixed with a further nine parts of inert substance and successed as before, producing a 2x potency. This would appear to be equivalent to a 100:1 dilution, but actually the two-stage 10:1 dilution produces a subtly different therapeutic effect.

By continuing the process homoeopathic dilutions can be prepared of increasing potencies (though this is not necessarily a measure of their potentiality, as will be seen later). Thus a 6x potency will correspond to a dilution of one part in a million which would appear to leave an utterly negligible trace of the original substance, though it can be detected by the sophisticated methods of modern chemistry. Yet some subtle influence remains. Scientific investigation, in fact, has provided various examples of tangible effects produced by such microdoses. For instance, it has been found that thyroxin can influence the growth of tadpoles in dilutions of one part in five million.

The preparation of these medicaments is now a highly specialized art. The initial substances are simple chemical or herbal compounds, diluted with appropriate inert matter which may be solid (e.g. sugar of milk) or liquid (e.g. alcohol and/or water), vigorously shaken at each stage as already described. For some purposes even greater dilutions are used. Thus by mixing the original substance with 99 parts of inert matter a range of centesimal potencies can be prepared, designated 1c, 2c etc., while occasionally thousand-fold dilutions are used (1M, 10M etc.). It is unnecessary to go into details here, for suitable preparations are available of any required potency from specialist dispensers, such as Nelson's of Duke Street, London, W1, to the prescription of the practitioner. For psionic analysis appropriate preparations are often derived from organic material such as amino acids or protein.

It was the discovery that the power of his remedies was not only maintained, but even enhanced, by these dilutions which led Hahnemann to suggest that their proven efficacy arose from some non-physical form of energy content. This is, in fact, the secret of the process, for the method of potentizing which he adopted appears to provide a progressive distillation of the essential energy. Why this should be so is not clear. The vigorous succussion may have some influence on the molecular structure, but a more likely explanation would seem to be that while in the original substance a large part of the inherent energy has to be manifest in material form, this requirement is progressively reduced by the successive dilutions, thereby preserving a relatively increased proportion of the etheric energy.

Whatever the reason, it is found in practice that the curative action depends not only on the medicament itself, but is determined to a marked extent by its potency—which is why the term is used in preference to dilution. This has, indeed, been demonstrated by tests on the germination of seeds subjected to homoeopathic nutrition, which showed that optimum growth was achieved with certain potencies, while others produced a retarding effect.

Hence it is necessary when prescribing a remedy to specify not only the substance, but its potency; and since it is a basic tenet of homoeopathy that the treatment is related to the individual and not merely to the ailment the prescription is essentially dependent on an understanding of the patient. This necessarily involves the intuition of the practitioner to a greater extent than with conventional allopathic treatment (though even here a good physician will use his intuitive faculties). Hence a certain amount of exploration is usually required to discover the appropriate remedy. Even then, since the treatment is concerned with the correction of imbalances in the vital energies, a certain time may elapse before it takes effect, which does not accord with the popular demand for instant cure.

Allopathic remedies can often provide a useful and rapid alleviation of distress, but these should be regarded as no more than palliatives providing a temporary respite while the body exercises its inherent curative power. If the symptoms persist it becomes necessary to seek, and endeavour to remedy, the underlying causes, and here homoeopathic (and psionic) techniques can be of great assistance. There is, indeed, great danger in the continued use of drugs without proper understanding, of which I have had unfortunate personal experience, for at one time my wife was prescribed a course of drugs for migraine. These achieved an apparent cure, but the treatment was continued far too long, producing a distressing condition of endogenous depression, which required psychiatric treatment. Yet the medical textbooks clearly state that prolonged use of these drugs will produce exactly this effect, of which one would have expected the practitioner to be well aware. This is a typical example of the treatment of the symptoms, rather than the patient, and I have since always checked with my pendulum any drugs prescribed for either of us, to make sure that they are not inimical to the life force.

The situation is made worse by the vast array of supposedly innocuous drugs which are available without medical prescription.

These are taken indiscriminately by the public, and can prove addictive. There is no awareness of the fact that the true function of a medicament is to assist the body to heal itself, and since the supply of these remedies is a highly lucrative business the manufacturers do not go out of their way to enjoin moderation in their use beyond cautionary statements that it is dangerous to exceed the prescribed dose, which the general public does not take very seriously.

We are not concerned here with the details of homoeopathic practice, which is already extensively documented. One school of thought relies solely on medication using uniform doses of high potency, but the more usual approach today relates the potency to the individual requirements. Moreover, it regards the technique as augmenting orthodox knowledge. So that given a proper understanding, conventional remedies can be used with advantage for the relief of suffering pending the response of the body to the treatment of the underlying causes; and this will include purely mechanical techniques such as osteopathy or surgery.

As already mentioned, the real basis of homoeopathy, and indeed of any true method of healing, is the treatment of the patient rather than the symptoms, which was the fundamental principle of Hahnemann's philosophy. Hence the medicaments of the extensive *Materia Medica* are not regarded as specifics against a particular disease, but are assessed in terms of their ability to restore the vital harmony of the individual. The same principles apply to the techniques of psionic medicine, as we shall see; and there is an important corollary of the technique which is that as and when the medicaments produce an amelioration of the conditions it becomes necessary to re-examine the *patient*, and modify the treatment to enable the restoration to be continued.

It is evident, however, that the successful development of this essential understanding necessarily involves a considerable element of intuition, which is usually dismissed as unscientific. This is a complete misconception, for the intuitive faculty depends on the use of the paranormal senses, which can be cultivated; and as we shall see later when discussing extra-sensory perception, the interpretations provided by the paranormal senses are not haphazard, but conform to a reasoning of a superior quality.

They provide, in fact, a more conscious understanding, using the word in its true meaning of 'knowing all together'. To be aware of the unmanifest causes of observed phenomena clearly involves an entirely superior quality of understanding which augments, and in fact embraces, the ordinary sense-based knowledge. It has a certain quality of compassion, quite different from mere sympathy—which can only distract one's judgment. It is the exercise of an innate flair (which the dictionary defines as an instinctive selection of what is excellent), and while this can be developed with practice, it can be greatly assisted by the techniques of psionic medicine which can provide quantitative assessments of aberrant conditions from which the nature, and potency, of the appropriate remedy can be determined with precision.

The practical details will emerge as we proceed but we must first inquire more closely into the nature of the disturbances of the vital energy pattern which are the cause of the clinical symptoms. These Hahnemann called *miasms*, which he regarded as hereditary. Laurence, however, has established that there are also contemporary miasms, as we shall see in the next chapter. These are acquired during the lifetime of the individual, and are perhaps better described as residual or acquired toxins, constituting a kind of hangover in the etheric body. We shall see that either type will respond to treatment designed to restore the vital harmony.

Chapter 5

Miasms and Toxins

Although Hahnemann formulated the principles of homoeopathy in his *Organon der rationelle Heilkunde* as early as 1810, when he was 55, it was not until much later that he conceived the idea of miasms. He had compiled an extensive list of preparations which had been systematically observed to produce certain symptoms in healthy volunteers. He then began to apply these medicaments equally systematically to actual sufferers from these complaints, and achieved over the years an encouraging measure of success, which confirmed his belief that, properly administered, like cures like.

However, he found that the treatment appeared not to be fully effective against certain types of chronic disease. He observed that these diseases, even after being repeatedly and successfully treated by the then-known homoeopathic remedies, continually reappeared in a more or less modified form, with a yearly increase in disagreeable symptoms. He came to the conclusion that these symptoms were really the result of some unknown 'primitive malady' and he devoted the last eleven years of his long and fruitful life to the attempt to elucidate this hidden cause.

Let us try to follow his intuition. It was a fundamental tenet of his belief that the presence of disease implied a departure from the harmonious relationship of the vital energies; so that the prescription of homoeopathic remedies which themselves contained the appropriate energies could restore the balance and so effect a cure. This is broadly true, and is in fact the basis of the treatment. But he came to realize that a superficial interpretation of the results contained an inherent fallacy, namely the assumption that it was the disease, resulting from some inimical life condition, which was disturbing the vital harmony, whereas it seemed more likely, particularly with chronic conditions, that it was the departure from true harmony which was producing the disease.

This reinforces the idea put forward some two centuries earlier by Thomas Sydenham, usually regarded as the father of British medicine, that illness is itself a form of cure, an attempt by the body to rectify some derangement of the vital force.

Hahnemann therefore postulated the existence of what he called *miasms*. These were disturbances of the unseen pattern of vital energy which, in his words, caused parasitical ramifications to spread through the human organism and grow therein. He suggested that there were three basic types of miasm, two of which were specific, namely Syphilis and Sycosis, while the third, which he called Psora, was a hydra-headed miasm responsible for a variety of conditions.

This miasmic theory of chronic disease has never gained adequate recognition in orthodox circles, mainly because it is not understood. The idea, indeed, has become quite incorrectly interpreted even by the Homoeopathic Faculty, which defines miasms as 'specific parasitic infection by micro-organisms'. But this is confusing effect with cause, and to equate miasms with microbes is a misinterpretation of Hahnemann's intuitive insight. He was unable to formulate his ideas precisely in terms of the limited medical and scientific knowledge of his time, but the developments of biochemistry and dowsing have made possible a new and very practical basis of understanding.

Let us examine the idea in relation to the concept of the etheric body discussed earlier. This we have seen to be a pattern of unmanifest force-fields through which the transit of consciousness creates the successive phenomena of the physical body. This materialization will take place in accordance with specific and established laws, of which today we have a very detailed knowledge. We know the body to be a structure of cells, assembled in highly specialized groups, each having their own genetic code, directed by an overall co-ordinating intelligence which sustains the remarkable pattern of bodily functions.

The behaviour of this structure is subject to the laws of physical cause and effect which operate throughout the phenomenal world. Many bodily disorders can be ascribed to observable physical causes, and orthodox medical treatment is based on a similar pattern of observed physical cause and effect. Yet there are cases in which the cause is not so readily discernible, and one has to adopt palliatives, which may not be fully effective.

The concept of the etheric body introduces a different dimension into the structure. If one regards the physical body as a progressive interpretation in the phenomenal world of an existing pattern of possibilities in the unmanifest realm, it is evident that the material structure can be affected by influences of a superior order, while still being subject to the laws of physical cause and effect; and any derangement of this underlying energy pattern will create effects in the material body which cannot be interpreted, or treated, in terms of physical cause.

These derangements are the miasms of Hahnemann's vision. They reside in the etheric body and are thus not able to be detected by physical means, though their clinical effects are; and for this reason they have long been unrecognized by orthodox medicine. Yet practical experience has now established that they can be detected, and if necessary modified, by the exercise of the paranormal senses. For over a century this has been a purely intuitive skill, but the techniques of psionic medicine have enabled these faculties to be developed with scientific precision, thereby providing an effective treatment of formerly incurable chronic conditions.

How do these miasms arise? It will be evident that since the etheric body is the unmanifest counterpart of the physical body there will be a relationship between them which can operate in both directions, so that if in the course of time in the material world some extraneous happening, such as an infection, disturbs the harmony of the physical body, this must be accompanied by a corresponding derangement of the etheric body. But whereas in the further passage of time the physical functioning may be restored, the disturbance in the etheric body remains. This constitutes a miasm, as a kind of permanent (but not necessarily irremediable) scar.

The presence of such miasms causes a general weakening of the vital harmony, which creates a predisposition to a variety of physical disorders with which the inherent intelligence of the body may be unable to cope, leading to the development of chronic symptoms. Moreover, and even more significantly, since these aberrations occur within the timeless realm of the etheric world, their influence extends beyond the individual life-span; so that, working backwards, a patient may be affected by miasms created in his immediate ancestry.

These are Hahnemann's hereditary miasms. They transcend the purely physical patterns of heredity, for although much is now known about genetic codes and their transference from parent to offspring, these are merely the logical development in physical terms of underlying causes which operate within the fabric of the unmanifest realm; and it is because this superior world is not subject to the laws of passing time that it is possible, as Laurence has proved, to detect and correct miasms which have originated in what we regard as the past.

As mentioned earlier, however, similar aberrations in the etheric body can be created by illnesses during the lifetime of the individual. These can be called acquired miasms, though Laurence prefers to refer to them as residual or acquired toxins. The two main hereditary miasms are those of syphilis and tuberculosis. The acquired toxins are derived primarily from the infections of childhood, particularly measles, whooping cough and chicken pox, all of which are today amenable to treatment and hence regarded as of minor importance. But many such infections can develop miasmic aberrations which may lie dormant for many years before producing symptoms which appear quite unrelated to the original trouble; and the residual toxins of influenza, staphylococcus aureus, and some forms of b. coli can produce chronic symptoms later in life.

In an address to the British Society of Dowsers in September 1966 Dr Aubrey Westlake said:

> In a recent series of sixty consecutive cases, mostly chronic, the most common and undiagnosed cause of the condition was found to be the T.B. miasm. There were thirty-eight such cases out of the sixty; well over half. . . . The effect of this miasm is protean to an almost incredible extent. Dr. Laurence has listed a variety of ailments in which this miasm was found to be the fundamental underlying cause, and which can be cured or greatly helped by its elimination. The list includes asthma, eczema, hay fever, allergy conditions, chronic sinusitis, and chronic pharyngeal or laryngeal trouble, migraines, mental illness of various kinds including retardation

and subnormality, various abdominal symptoms, enuresis, heart symptoms, mucous colitis, varicose veins and arterial degeneration, diabetes, Hodgkin's disease and leukaemia.

A most important effect of the T.B. miasm is that it undoubtedly renders the patient much more liable to retain the toxins of acquired diseases in the system, of which measles is one of the most important. It has recently been reported in the medical press that encephalitis may be a complication or sequel to measles. Evidence of this has often appeared in psionic analysis. It also seems likely that the T.B. miasm may be an important factor in the development of carcinoma in later life. Carcinoma is not a separate entity, but a gradual build up of toxins, at least as a general rule, with some extra and often long continued toxaemia, such as smoking, finally precipitating the conversion to malignant disease. In the analysis of causes of cancer, the residual toxins of T.B. and measles only too often appear.

It is of interest to note that the existence of miasmic influences has recently been confirmed by orthodox medical science (though not under this name). A news item in the American press in March 1969, headed 'Many ills related to Smouldering Virus', read as follows:

WASHINGTON (AP)—United States government scientists reported yesterday that a breakthrough in virus research may shed some light on the causes of a wide variety of ills, ranging from some forms of cancer to maladies like multiple sclerosis and Parkinson's disease.

The breakthrough suggests, they reported, that a host of still-unsolved maladies may be due to 'smouldering' viruses left over from some common infection early in life, such as measles.

The development was reported by scientists of the National Institutes of Health. It concerned the isolation—after almost four years of research—of a virus suspected of being the cause of a rare and mysterious brain disease that annually strikes between 100 and 200 Americans of high school or early college age, always fatally.

The virus, isolated from brain tissue of a youthful victim, turned out to be identical with the virus long known to cause common measles.

The real explanation, of course, has been missed, for the virus is the effect rather than the cause. Yet these findings lend support to the idea of Hahnemann's 'primitive malady', and it is only a small step to postulate that this originates in a superior realm, not manifest to the senses, for which there is increasing evidence not only in the medical field but in the field of parapsychology in general. As the ranks of orthodoxy begin to accept this idea, and avail themselves of the scientific use of psionic analysis, many intractable problems will become capable of solution.

We shall deal later with the methods used to detect and treat these miasms by psionic techniques; and the case histories quoted later provide clear and practical evidence of the existence of these normally unsuspected causes. In a paper entitled 'Knowing and affecting by extra-sensory means' read to the Medical Society for the Study of Radiesthesia in October 1962, Dr Laurence says:

> The baffling characteristic of these miasms, and one that renders them so difficult to demonstrate to the orthodox, is the fact that there is no recognized clinical or laboratory test for their existence—hence, ipso facto, they must be purely mythical!
>
> For instance, actual syphilis can be inherited and give positive Wassermann or Kahn tests, but a syphilitic miasm or toxicosis can also be inherited which will afford no such tests and can only be detected by psionic methods and which may produce symptoms completely baffling unless you have the causal clue.
>
> Another, and much more common miasm to be passed on is of the tubercular type, the results of which are protean in character to a most extraordinary extent, both physical and mental. There is accumulating evidence that diabetes is generally, if not always, due to an inherited tubercular miasm.
>
> An interesting point is that people with this inherited taint never seem to develop actual clinical tuberculosis. The miasm seems to act as an immunising agent, but in view of the wide-spread prevalence of active tuberculosis in the past the frequent appearance of this particular miasm today is not surprising.

Laurence draws a clear distinction between physical and etheric predisposition. The former is well known in medical practice as diathesis, which is defined in Stedman's Medical Dictionary as 'a constitutional state predisposing to any disease or group of diseases'. But while such conditions are clinically observable they frequently arise from miasms in the etheric body, which one has to recognize as existing simultaneously with the physical symptoms. It is tempting to the doctor trained to recognize and treat specific diseases to seek direct correspondences with Hahnemann's miasms; but this does not necessarily accord with his intuition or intention. Dr Herbert A. Roberts, a distinguished American homoeopath, possibly recognized this when he summarized the character of the miasmic stigmata quite simply. The tendency of the syphilitic taint, he suggests, is ulcerative. That of sycosis is infiltrative and congestive, leading to deposits and tumour formation, the term deriving from the Greek word for a fig, or more correctly in the adjectival form 'swollen like a fig'; whilst the action of psora relates to functional imbalance.

This suggests that the miasms are fundamentally related to the expression of certain forces acting on matter; in this case living matter. A force moving centripetally towards a centre produces consolidation. Its opposite, moving centrifugally, results in expansion, whilst the force that reconciles the two opposing forces involves a mediating rhythmic activity. One can thus relate the first force to the processes of assimilation, the second to diffusion and elimination, and the third to circulatory activity in the broadest sense of the word.

Disordered assimilation would seem therefore to relate to the sycotic miasm in that deposits, congestion and tumour formation occur in excess of that normal to the organic formatory process. Disordered diffusion or eliminatory functions in cells, tissues and organs would result from the syphilitic miasm and the ulcerative tendency would arise. Psora would give rise to a disordered rhythmic function at all organic levels, which would account for the widespread variations of the effects of this miasm.

In practice there is usually more than one influence at work so that the issue is not nearly so clear-cut as the above would suggest. But there may be a dominance of one or another which affects the situation significantly. Carl Upton has suggested that since the dynamic energy involved in the life of the cell stems from the nucleus and is reflected in the activity of the cell body, then changes in intensity of nucleic energy may constitute the first material stage in the production of clinical symptoms. Such changes, he believes, are brought about by the etheric imbalance induced by miasms, acquired toxins and other agencies capable of producing etheric stress.

A persistent increase in intensity of nucleic energy could be associated with the sycotic miasm; and this would result in reactions in the cell body to contain this—namely, a condensation. On the other hand, the syphilitic miasm would be associated with a decrease of intensity of nucleic cell energy and consequent loss of tone of the cell body, leading to ultimate disintegration.

Psora would affect the mediating functional balance normally existing to maintain the functional integrity and purpose of the cell and would thus be likely to accentuate the effects of imbalance of the organic components that may already be present due to other miasms.

A cell that is subject to intense nucleic stimulation may well be the cell which manifests abnormal mitotic activity and division, with corresponding consolidation leading to tumour formation; especially if functional balance is disturbed in relation to an existing sycotic miasm. The opposite would apply in the case of loss of nucleic intensity. Atrophy, malformation, paralysis and psychotic manifestation could well be the result if psoric imbalance is superimposed on the syphilitic miasm.

It is perhaps pertinent to suggest that since the psoric factor is directly related to functional activity and is neither a component organically of nucleus or cell body, that it is in some way related to the emotional forces which play upon the organism. If this is so then one may well have to take these into account when studying the effects of psora-creating influences which are referred to in conventional homoeopathy as 'mentals'.

Upton sees here a certain analogy with the operation of conventional nuclear physics. In a nuclear explosion the devastation caused by the heat and blast is clearly evident. Less immediately apparent is the effect of the so-called 'fall-out', the insidious action of which may persist long after the superficial damage has been cleared and rebuilding has taken place, and which has destructive effects at much more subtle levels of matter: witness, for example, the effects on living tissue over generations. It is naturally tempting to ask whether it is not a biological nuclear explosion that occurs in acute infectious illness, the cell nuclei being affected and leading to local and repairable cell damage characteristic of acute disease processes on the one hand, but accompanied by a much more subtle damage to the etheric body —the effect of a biological 'fall-out'.

Furthermore, it is well known that the period of radioactive decay—customarily measured in terms of the 'half-life'—varies widely with different elements, ranging from a few minutes to hundreds of years. A similar effect appears to apply to biological fall-out. It is known in psionic medicine that according to the nature of the infecting organism so the period of persistence of the etheric effect varies. Syphilis and tuberculosis, for example, produce a fall-out which persists over several generations; and this it would seem is what places them in the category of miasms. Minor infections on the other hand persist for relatively short periods from several months to a few years, again according to the nature of the organism involved. But in any event the duration always transcends the period of the acute physical changes of orthodox clinical diagnosis. Later clinical effects over the period of the etheric imbalance are not usually recognized as part of the same episode, either because they differ in character or because they take some chronic form.

It is relevant here to note that etheric imbalances do not arise only from conventional infections but can be produced by normally unsuspected influences in the environment which are inimical to the human organism. The most important of these is the prevalent use of aluminium utensils both for cooking and in the preparation of processed foods. This has a deleterious influence which does not arise from any chemical interaction, but from the absorption by the food of intrinsic energies in the aluminium which are not compatible with bodily harmony.

This poisoning is not recognized by orthodox practice, but its influence is very widespread. Dr H. Tomlinson, in his book *The Divination of Disease*, deals with it at some length. He maintains that it causes imbalance of the ductless glands, and is responsible for a wide variety of ailments including duodenal and gastric ulcers, liver and gall bladder complaints, rectal diseases and cancer, all of which are increasingly prevalent today. Conventional chemotherapy can provide some alleviation, but does not treat the cause and so is only a palliative.

The prolonged absorption of this inimical energy produces aberrations in the etheric body, mainly acquired but often inherited, which can only be properly treated by homoeopathic methods. They can be very rapidly diagnosed by psionic analysis, by which the appropriate remedy can be assessed with precision, though some time may be required to rid the body of these insidious poisons.

Aluminium is not the only metal which contains noxious energy, though it is by far the most important because it is so widely used in the preparation of food; but any element which is not found naturally in the body will have similar effects, mercury and lead being the most common. These noxious influences, in fact, are the unsuspected cause of many ills, some specific, some resulting merely in a general lowering of vitality.

It is evident, therefore, that the pattern of health is influenced by a variety of unsuspected miasms and residual toxins, some deep-seated, producing chronic illness, others less severe which the intelligence of the body endeavours to correct itself. The significance of psionic medicine lies in its ability to assist this inherent faculty by the scientific location and correction of the disturbances in the underlying fabric of vital energy.

Chapter 6

The Unitary Theory of Disease

It was the conviction that true medicine was concerned with causes rather than clinical symptoms that prompted George Laurence to stretch his mind beyond the limits of ordinary acceptance. He began to investigate unconventional techniques, not from a purely theoretical standpoint, but as a method of reinforcing his well-established orthodox knowledge. But with a characteristic blend of caution and intuition he did not pin his faith to any one system, believing that all these methods were complementary facets of an underlying truth. Hence if we are to follow his quest we must also consider a variety of aspects of causal medicine, which may at first appear to be unconnected, but which will ultimately be seen to be integrated within the overall pattern.

Laurence acknowledges the influence of three great thinkers in his search for the truth. The first of these was Samuel Hahnemann, whose concept of illness as resulting from disturbance of the vital energy corresponded with Laurence's intuitive intimations of reality—a concept which we have already discussed in some detail in the two preceding chapters. The acceptance of these ideas is necessarily dependent on the understanding that the physical body is neither the whole, nor even the most important part, of a man (or woman), being simply a representation in terms of the ordinary senses of a much larger and comprehensive entity; and his thinking in this direction was influenced by the ideas of Rudolf Steiner, whose concept of the etheric world confirmed the possibility of influences and causes of a superior order, and whose notion of 'Formative Forces' provided a further reinforcement of the emerging pattern.

At this stage he came into contact with his third source of inspiration in the person of J. E. R. McDonagh FRCS, with whom he had a number of discussions. McDonagh had been pursuing the idea that all disease arose from a derangement of the vital energies in the body. These he believed to be responsible for the formation of proteins, which are the essential building blocks of all living matter, so that any disturbance of the vital harmony caused a corresponding aberration in the protein production. Hence he maintained that there was only one basic disease, which arose from some imbalance in the protein structure. The clinical symptoms, whatever their nature and classification, are merely evidence of malfunction of some part of the intricate mechanisms of the body, arising entirely from an aberration of the protein. So although these symptoms can be studied in great detail, and the conditions partially ameliorated by palliative techniques of various kinds, no real cure is possible unless the underlying protein imbalance can be redressed.

The extent of this aberration determines the seriousness of the disorder and McDonagh suggested that malignant disease is the result of an extreme degree of protein imbalance and hence is a constitutional malady and not just a local disturbance.

This is a very simplified statement of what is known as the Unitary Theory of Disease, a very significant concept which is by no means universally accepted. We shall discuss it in more detail shortly, but it is evident that it provides an important link between the etheric and the physical worlds. If the primary cause of illness is a disharmony of the vital energies, one can understand that this can be manifest in physical terms as an imbalance of the protein structure, resulting in the clinical symptoms of disease. Laurence intuitively recognized the practical possibilities of this concept and was able by patient experiment to utilize it in developing the integrated technique of diagnosis and treatment which has become the basis of psionic medicine.

McDonagh's ideas were ahead of his time, unacceptable to orthodox materialism which found his detailed formulations difficult, and even fanciful. Yet his basic concept is entirely compatible with modern scientific thought which, as we have seen, regards matter as a local condensation of an all-pervading energy pattern. Science affirms that physical matter is an assemblage of molecules which are themselves ordered combinations of fundamental chemical elements called atoms. But this is only the beginning of the story, for these atoms in their turn are structures of sub-microscopic electrical particles called electrons revolving round a central nucleus in a kind of miniature solar system; and it is the number and disposition of these orbiting electrons which determines the distinguishing characteristics of the hundred-odd chemical elements. The simplest element is the gas called hydrogen, the lightest of all elements, which has only one orbiting electron. Carbon has six, nitrogen seven and oxygen eight. Phosphorus, an essential constituent of cellular structure, has fifteen, while the atoms of very heavy elements such as lead may contain more than eighty electrons.

It is irrelevant here to discuss atomic structure in detail, though its patterns are of a fascinating elegance. The orbiting electrons are not arranged in haphazard order, but occupy successive shells corresponding to specific energy levels. Each shell can contain up to eight electrons (except the innermost which can only hold two) and the chemical affinity between different elements, which creates the wide range of compounds in nature, is based on the fulfilment of this quota of eight. Thus sodium, which contains only one electron in its outermost shell, combines very readily with chlorine, which has seven outer electrons, to produce a molecule of sodium chloride (more familiarly known as common salt); and the whole structure of chemical compounds is based on the grouping of appropriate elements—often more than two—which between them complete this octave pattern.

The familiar materials of the ordinary environment are aggregations of relatively simple molecules, natural and artificial, which arrange themselves in ordered structures having specific properties of which the chemist or the engineer makes appropriate use. Living matter, however, uses a more elaborate structure in which a relatively small number of elements form themselves into units which then repeat themselves to produce long chain-like molecules containing several hundred links; and these form the basis of the organisms called cells of which living matter is composed.

We shall discuss this later, but in the immediate context there is an aspect of the subject which is of profound significance, namely that all these structures are of limited duration. We are accustomed to the idea that living organisms have a finite lifetime, which varies with the species. For man, the average life span is some eighty years, but this is a macroscopic assessment, for during this period the cells of the body are continually dying, to be replaced by new ones, the lifetime of the average cell being of the order of a day. But these cells are themselves complex assemblies of molecules constructed of atoms; and these in turn are patterns of sub-microscopic electrons which by ordinary standards are utterly impermanent. Scientific evidence indicates that the lifetime of an electron is of the order of 1/10,000th of a second. It is impossible to pinpoint an electron. All that can be said is that there is evidence that it was there a moment ago; and the lifetime of some of the constituents of the nucleus of the atom is measured in fractions of a microsecond.

We live indeed in a world of illusion in which the very building blocks of our materials have an almost negligible existence, requiring continuous replacement. The replenishment of the cells of the body is assumed to be undertaken by the ordinary processes of nourishment, directed by the intelligence of the body, but it is evident that this is an altogether too superficial view, since the raw materials of the atoms themselves are being continually replenished by some much more subtle form of nourishment.

In terms of ordinary sense-based intelligence these more refined implications are unnecessary. It is possible to cope quite adequately with material problems by the application of conventional knowledge. But we have seen that this knowledge is of a strictly limited character, and particularly in its medical aspects falls far short of a true understanding. If we are to surmount this barrier it is necessary to relate our thinking to the concepts of the real world, and specifically to the pattern of the etheric realm in which the true causes and relationships exist.

We saw in chapter 3 that the etheric world is a fabric of (unmanifest) relationships within which the interplay of influences creates the various effects which the senses interpret as the matter/energies of the physical world; and since the senses only respond to changes of condition it is evident that this cannot be a static process but must be of a dynamic character involving repeating cycles of growth and decay. Hence the physical world is not a permanent crystallization of the etheric fabric, but is continuously being created by rhythmic condensations of the etheric force-field in successively more complex form.

This is an unfamiliar idea by conventional standards, though it is entirely consistent with esoteric cosmology, which regards the universe as a living entity animated by a continual flow and return of energy, called in Hindu philosophy the Breath of Brahma; but even in material terms it has been suggested on the basis of scientific evidence that the physical universe is being continuously created out of the void.

This was the idea which McDonagh endeavoured to develop in support of his Unitary Theory of Disease. He formulated the concept in considerable detail, notably in a series of writings on the nature of disease, but because this involved new directions of thought, in advance of accepted ideas, his theories met with little recognition, and even provoked hostility. Moreover, this very detail tended to obscure the essential simplicity of his vision, namely that it was possible for these ordered processes to become deranged and that it was these aberrations from the norm which produced the symptoms of disease.

It was this aspect of the idea which Laurence intuitively recognized as providing the integrating factor in his study of the imbalance of vital energy and which he was then able to apply to provide a practical system of therapy. How this can be achieved will be discussed in more detail later, but to understand the possibilities we must review in simple terms the basis of McDonagh's theory. Briefly, he postulates a primordial 'activity' (which we have called the etheric force-field) from which the matter-energies of the physical world are formed by a sequence of pulsations in an evolutionary spiral. The first stage creates the sub-atomic particles—the protons and electrons of physics—of almost negligible life span, but continually replenished.

The second cycle is concerned with the integration of these particles into atoms, forming three distinct (unequal) groups performing specific functions which he calls radiation, attraction and storage. This is broadly in line with orthodox chemistry, the metallic elements playing a predominantly active role, which can be regarded as the radiative function, while the basic elements exercise the attractive function and the inert gases the storage function.

The third cycle involves the formation of simple molecules and their arrangement in the crystalline structures which constitute the basis of inorganic matter. Here again the compounds, according to their nature, exercise one of the three specific functions, which determines their quality in the overall chemical structure.

There then follows a fourth cycle concerned with the more elaborate molecular structures of so-called organic compounds. These include the colloids, such as albumen, and the amino-acids which are the building blocks of protein, the essential constituent of living matter. There appears at this stage to be an infusion of vital energy—possibly the *Vis Medicatrix Naturae*—which permits the molecules to exercise all the three primary functions in an appropriate degree, instead of only one as with the inorganic compounds.

From this develops a fifth cycle in which the proteins are elaborated into the various interdependent structures of the vegetable world, followed by the sixth cycle concerned with the requirements of the animal kingdom in which the proteins are diversified into the tissues and organs of the body.

According to McDonagh, life is sustained by the continuous pulsation of vital energy in the essential proteins, each of which must provide an appropriate and harmonious exercise of the functions of radiation, attraction and storage. What this implies in practical terms will be discussed later, but it is possible to understand that if this essential rhythm is disturbed by some extraneous influence—such as the miasms of Hahnemann's philosophy—this will produce a condition of disease, accompanied by clinical symptoms of varying severity.

This is the basis of McDonagh's contention that there is only one disease, which arises from the protein in the blood being so affected that it can no longer exercise its proper functions of attracting nourishment (not necessarily physical), storing the energy appropriately and radiating it to the tissues and organs. The clinical effects can vary from the acute to the chronic, and may to some extent be alleviated by chemotherapy, but no real cure can be provided until the aberration of the protein has been diagnosed and a harmonious balance restored.

It is, of course, in the practical assessment of these aberrations that the principal difficulty lies, for the validity of any theory can only be established by experimental verification; and this would appear to depend to an even greater extent than homoeopathy on the intuition of the practitioner, which is why the idea has not received more acceptance.

Yet as has been said earlier, intuition is not such a haphazard process as is popularly supposed, being actually an exercise of the paranormal senses which can be both scientific and precise. Hence before discussing the concept of protein imbalance in detail we must consider more specifically the nature of the extra-sensory faculties, and how they may be cultivated and applied.

Chapter 7

Extra-sensory Perception

Several references have been made in the preceding chapters to the existence of paranormal senses which are responsible for the faculty usually called intuition; and since the diagnosis and treatment of the underlying causes of disease involve the scientific use of these faculties it is desirable to discuss the nature and possibilities of these paranormal senses in some detail.

We have already established that the physical world of everyday experience is only an interpretation, by a strictly limited range of senses, of a superior but unmanifest pattern of possibilities which contains the real causes and relationships which govern the events and experiences of life. We are, however, provided with a range of additional senses which respond to impressions of a different quality, which are not detected by the conventional senses. These are called the paranormal senses, meaning that they exist side by side with the normal physical senses. There are people in whom these latent faculties are unusually developed, which tends to create the belief that they are in some way abnormal. But this is incorrect, for these additional senses are part of man's normal equipment, but are unused and therefore dormant.

With our preoccupation with material phenomena we take the physical senses completely for granted, and fail to realize that we have had to be educated to interpret their responses. A similar education is necessary to exercise the paranormal senses, but this we do not normally find necessary because we can cope quite adequately with the world of facts by the processes of logical reasoning.

Nevertheless, we have a cursory awareness of these paranormal responses, which produces what is customarily called sensitivity. We instinctively like or dislike people or places. We recognize that certain situations are right, without being able to say why. All too often we dismiss these feelings as illogical or superstitious, but they are actually responses to the real relationships of the situation which are understood by the superior intelligence of the paranormal senses.

There is abundant evidence of the existence of these paranormal senses, usually in their more spectacular manifestations in the form of telepathy and clairvoyance; and of recent years there has been established an accepted science of parapsychology which is concerned with the study of these phenomena. The pioneer of these investigations was J. B. Rhine of Duke University, California. He embarked on a painstaking series of tests using five cards bearing distinctive emblems which were selected in random order, while the subject in a separate room was required to 'guess' which card was being presented. Some subjects proved more sensitive than others, but the overall result was that the average proportion of successes was significantly greater than would be expected from the statistical laws of chance.

Since then there has been considerable investigation of psi phenomena, as they are called, covering not only extra-sensory perception, popularly abbreviated to e.s.p., but also a wide range of associated phenomena such as telepathy, clairvoyance, precognition and psychokinesis (the ability to influence physical objects or events at a distance). It is accepted that such possibilities exist, and it is assumed that they are in some way functions of the mind. But the results are only partially conclusive because it is assumed that the mind is directed by an intelligence of the same order as that which provides the translations of the physical senses.

This is a fundamental error, for the mind is not part of the physical body, but is an immaterial entity directed by an intelligence of a superior and incommensurable order. This is a subject which I have discussed at length in my book *The Diary of a Modern Alchemist* which is concerned with the psychological relationships of the unmanifest world. It will suffice to note here that the paranormal senses cannot be understood in material terms. The ordinary senses are mechanisms which respond to impressions derived from the physical world; but we have seen that the influences in the etheric world create a variety of manifestations at the phenomenal level which are not detected by the physical senses, and it is to these additional stimuli that the paranormal senses respond.

A correct interpretation of the undoubted existence of this 'sixth sense' can only be provided by the acceptance of this concept. Nor is this a new idea, for over one hundred years ago the distinguished German chemist von Reichenbach, noted among other things for the discovery of creosote, postulated the existence of a universal fluid which he called Odyle. This he regarded as permeating the whole of nature, providing a medium for the transmission of what he called the *Vis Occulta*, which he considered to be responsible for many admitted 'imponderables', including the auras surrounding the body which can be discerned by sensitive subjects. The idea was far ahead of its time and was entirely rejected by the material science of the era, so that he died a disappointed man.

Yet one finds in the literature many similar concepts such as the Munia of Paracelsus, the Vital Fluid of the medieval alchemists, or the Prana of Indian philosophy; and Westlake has suggested that Reichenbach's 'odic force' is in fact the *Vis Medicatrix Naturae* mentioned earlier. All these concepts are consistent with the idea that the influences in the etheric world do not only create the familiar everyday phenomena, but are also responsible for a variety of manifestations to which the ordinary senses do not respond, but which are nevertheless part of the structure of the phenomenal world.

This provides a coherent, and scientific, understanding of the many observed effects which defy explanation in material terms. We need not discuss the mechanism in detail. It is sufficient for practical purposes to note that these intangible patterns can be detected by the paranormal senses and interpreted by the higher levels of the mind, which by their very nature can communicate with the etheric world.

If the paranormal senses were fully developed they would provide a complete understanding of the real causes and relationships in the phenomenal world. There are people who possess a certain natural sensitivity and who therefore display an unusual degree of intuition, though for most of us it is indifferently exercised. It is nevertheless a faculty which can be developed, once its existence is recognized.

In the medical context, the paranormal senses permit

communication with the intelligence of the body. This is of a higher order, directed by a part of the (non-physical) mind which has a complete understanding of the requirements of the organism. It is aware of any imbalances and aberrations, which it seeks to remedy with its own resources. This may be beyond its capacity in which case some external assistance may be required, but if this is to be effective it must be such as to assist, and not override, the innate intelligence of the body. This is well understood by the enlightened physician, though there are still far too many examples of medical arrogance.

How then can this latent faculty of intuition be developed? It is a matter of practice for, as mentioned earlier, the paranormal senses have to be educated. One has first to recognize the existence of this innate sensitivity, which we all possess in varying degree, and then strengthen it by increasing acknowledgment. Initially it may be necessary to rely on orthodox knowledge, but one begins to interpret this with greater understanding, based on the acceptance of a higher level of intelligence, with which one seeks to communicate.

Now fortunately there is an eminently practical way of establishing this communication, by the use of the technique known as dowsing. It has long been known that under suitable conditions the paranormal senses can create involuntary muscular influences which produce physical responses in some simple detecting device. The classic example is the forked twig of the water diviner or 'dowser'—a term derived from an old Cornish word meaning to strike. Such a device held in the hands with the end horizontal will, with practice, exhibit a pronounced downward (or upward) tilt when the operator passes over subterranean water. This is a very ancient art, used with great success by experienced dowsers; and its application is not confined to water divining, for it can be used to locate oil or metal deposits, or even archaeological remains. Its reactions, in fact, depend on the questions which the operator asks, as we shall see.

The forked rod is not the only form of detector. The early experiments in radiesthesia used a variety of devices, some of which have already been described, in order to obtain a tangible response to questions posed by the operator; and for many purposes, particularly in medical dowsing, a convenient detector is a simple pendulum consisting of a light bob on the end of a short length of thread or chain which is held in the hand over, or in association with, the object under investigation. It then begins to swing in a variety of ways which, with practice, will provide clear and unequivocal answers to questions in the mind of the operator. This is a well-established technique, which will be discussed in detail in the next chapter.

These phenomena are of established authenticity, and there are many reputable institutions such as the British Society of Dowsers, which are concerned with the scientific investigation and application of the art. The effects are clearly dependent on the exercise of some kind of extra-sensory perception, and this we have seen cannot be explained in terms of sense-based reasoning. Hence to understand them it is necessary to employ a measure of emotional conjecture.

The mind is customarily considered to be of a purely intellectual character; but this is a very superficial assumption, for the mind, which is the instrument of consciousness, is a much more comprehensive structure, and the intellectual function, which is concerned with the logical reasoning of the ordinary senses, is only a small part of its activity. Its totality includes the superior understanding of the relationships in the unmanifest realm, and it is this which directs the paranormal senses, which thus have an emotional quality. Now it is well known that feelings produce corresponding physical responses, so that one can understand that the operations of the paranormal senses create small involuntary muscular tensions which influence the behaviour of a pendulum or other interpretative device.

It will be evident that if the indications are to be reliable the reactions must be involuntary, and it is easy to override them by voluntary direction. Hence it is essential to cultivate a passivity of mind which neither expects nor prejudges the answer, and this requires a certain amount of training, as is discussed in the next chapter. Nevertheless, experience proves that this facility is available, and can be cultivated to a much greater extent than is popularly believed.

It remains to consider how the paranormal senses can communicate with the relationships existing in the real world. Here one can be assisted by Swedenborg's concept of time-body. This again I have discussed in detail in the book mentioned earlier, but we can review the idea briefly in terms of what has already been postulated. We have seen that the appearances of the physical world are a translation of the successive manifestations in time of a superior, and relatively eternal fabric in the real world. This means that the progress of events in the phenomenal world leaves a permanent (though not unalterable) trace in the real world, which is called the time-body. All the events, and physical conditions, of life thus have their counterpart in the etheric world as a pattern which continues to exist when the finger of time has moved on, so that the transitory situations of life are merely a translation by the physical senses of a much greater and permanent entity in the real world.

This is a concept of enormously expanded potentialities. It not only confirms the idea previously mentioned that the physical body is only a small part of the real structure, but even more significantly, it is applicable to the whole of the phenomenal world, so that every object in the familiar world has its own time-body which extends in the realm of eternity far beyond its transitory appearance. Moreover, this time-body will include everything that has happened to it during its lifetime, which may be much longer than the human life span.

This is sometimes interpreted by saying that every object in nature contains its own intrinsic (intangible) vibrations; but this would seem to be an unnecessary complication. It is simpler to think in terms of time-body, which contains the whole history of the object, *and its associations*. This is an important corollary, for the etheric world, in which the time-body resides, is essentially a pattern of relationships, within which there are many connections which are not apparent to conventional observation. The paranormal senses, which are of a superior order, can respond to impressions emanating from any part of the time-body, and so assess the real causes and situations behind the physical manifestations.

It is thus possible to understand how information as to the real condition of a patient can be obtained from a blood spot or similar sample. The physical constitution of the sample is unimportant, its significance being that it establishes a link between the mind of the practitioner and the time-body of the patient; and hence its influence is not confined to the moment in time when it was originally supplied, but can continue to provide information about subsequent conditions.

This link between the mind of the dowser and the situation under examination is an essential requirement of the technique (which is why it cannot be mechanized). One has to hold in mind the patient, or situation, under consideration and then formulate a specific question, discarding utterly any preconceived notions, when a clear and unequivocal answer is obtained, if the question has been correctly framed.

The cultivation of this necessary passivity of mind involves considerable practice, coupled with a certain humility. One is, in effect, asking questions of the universe—but a universe of far greater intelligence and consciousness than one's own. It is said that the universe is fundamentally a structure of response to request, and will always give a faithful answer to questions put to it. But the quality of the answers is dependent upon the nature and precision of the request; and if this is couched in material terms, the answer will be of similar level.

(In parenthesis, one may note that all orthodox scientific development is a process of questioning, and if the answers are not what is expected it is because the question is wrong, and must be re-formulated; and psychologically many of the events of life are actually responses to requests which, in the main, we are not aware of having made.)

If one wishes to communicate with a superior level it is first necessary to acknowledge that a higher level exists. Then with a quiet mind, ignoring the clamour of habitual associations, it is possible to frame one's question; but as we shall see, this must be precise and unadulterated.

There is a wealth of literature on extra-sensory phenomena and any detailed discussion here would be inappropriate. However, this brief review of the possible mechanism of the paranormal faculties, and their application to dowsing, will serve to provide a background to the practical discussions which follow.

One of the aspects which is, at first, difficult to understand is the ability to communicate with a person, or a situation, at a distance, or in some other part of passing time. To appreciate this we must remember that the time-body contains a permanent record of the unmanifest pattern, including all its subtle interconnections with other time-bodies; and the quiet mind of the experienced dowser can communicate with any part of this real fabric, provided that he has some suitable sample to serve as a focus for his thoughts.

As a practical example of the extraordinary possibilities which exist we may refer to the practice of map dowsing, which is quite inexplicable in conventional terms. An experienced dowser can locate water or other deposits by using his pendulum on a map of the locality, subsequently confirming the indications by inspection of the actual site. This is particularly useful in archaeological research, where it is possible to examine the map of an area suspected of containing the buried remains of Roman or other civilizations. If this proves positive a local search is made, often with surprisingly accurate results.

Now while one can understand that the time-body of the original Roman villa or other structure continues to exist in the etheric world, including its subsequent history through the intervening centuries, its connection with a modern map seems more obscure. The map, of course, is a reproduction, maybe many times removed, of an actual survey of the site, and thereby contains a tenuous contact with the etheric pattern; but its main significance is that it serves as a focus for the mind of the dowser, whereby his paranormal senses can establish communication with the time-body of the actual locality.

This is an example of the subtle interconnections which exist in the etheric world. The time-body of an object or location is not confined to the physical entity but includes everything with which it has been connected throughout its existence. We often refer to a house as having a pleasant (or evil) 'atmosphere'. This intuitive feeling is an unconscious exercise of the paranormal sense, which is aware of the emotional influences of its former inhabitants. The stones of a cathedral are impregnated with the influences not only of the original masons but of the thousands of worshippers who have used it subsequently. Similarly the quality of any work of art or music is determined not merely by its creator but by all its subsequent history and experiences.

Psionic medicine is concerned with more immediate influences extending normally over a few generations only. Its significance lies in the fact that by the use of the normally dormant paranormal senses it is possible, practically and scientifically, to communicate with the time-body of a patient, and provide effective treatment, if necessary, of any aberrations disclosed.

Chapter 8

The Dowser's Pendulum

As has been said in the previous chapter, one of the most convenient forms of extra-sensory detector is the pendulum, which consists of a small weight or bob on the end of a cord. This will swing to and fro, like the pendulum of a clock, but if it is held in the hand it can be susceptible to paranormal influences which will affect its mode of oscillation, and so provide a basis of communication with the problem under investigation.

There are two forms of the device. One uses a suspension several feet in length and is therefore called the long pendulum. This is employed by some dowsers as an alternative to the conventional divining rod for prospecting and similar purposes, in which it has certain advantages. However, we are not concerned here with this kind of usage, which therefore need not be discussed. The alternative form, known as the short pendulum, is only a few inches in length and can conveniently be carried in the pocket. This is of much more widespread application, and the present discussion will be limited to this simpler type.

This short pendulum can be used in a variety of ways as an interrogating device. It consists of a small bob on the end of a thread or chain which is held lightly between the thumb and the first (or second) finger of the hand over an appropriate sample and is then mentally related to the problem under investigation. In due course it will begin to swing, which can take place in several ways, varying from a simple to-and-fro movement to a circular or gyratory motion, and the mode of its behaviour provides the answer to the dowser's question.

There are three basic forms of response, namely:

1 A simple to-and-fro oscillation, usually but not necessarily towards and away from the operator;

2 a rotatory or gyrating movement in a clockwise direction;
3 a gyration in an anticlockwise direction.

It is these movements, or combinations thereof, which provide the answers to the questions which are being posed by the dowser. There is no hard-and-fast rule, for the response differs in minor particulars for different operators, so that one has to find by experiment the pattern of one's individual response; but once this has been established, it will be found to be consistent.

The significant feature is that the pendulum will only react intelligibly to specific questions, formulated in the mind of the operator. As a very simple example, I have in front of me as I write a small nameplate of unknown composition. If I hold my pendulum over it, it will gyrate. If I now ask 'Is this made of steel?' the pendulum takes no notice. If I say 'Does it contain copper?' the pendulum at once begins to swing towards me, a reaction which I know from experience indicates yes. If I now ask 'Is copper the only material?' the pendulum continues to gyrate, saying no, but if I now postulate brass, which is an alloy of copper and zinc, it says yes.

This is a trivial example to illustrate how, once one has acquired the expertise, the pendulum will answer specific questions. It should be noted that it is a personal example, posed within the background of my own technical knowledge and therefore giving an answer valid for me in terms of that experience. Without this familiarity the reactions of the pendulum might be inconclusive, and even nonsense.

Hence it is essential to have an adequate knowledge of the subject under investigation, so that one can be aware of the possibilities, and pose intelligent questions. Given such a background the pendulum can be used to investigate much more subtle problems, and is in fact so used in psionic analysis, but in all cases it is necessary to be precisely aware of what question is being asked.

This is not as easy as it sounds for one's ordinary thinking is lamentably imprecise. A typical instance is the case of an inexperienced dowser who attempted to locate some buried drains in a recently-purchased field, without success. However, it transpired in a subsequent conversation that she had been looking for water, whereas the drains, being old, were almost certainly blocked and dry. By asking specifically, 'Are there any tile drains here?' positive indications were obtained which were later confirmed by actual digging.

This precise formulation is evidently still more essential in the investigation of medical problems which requires not only clear thinking but a sound background of orthodox knowledge and experience.

We shall see later how the pendulum is used in psionic analysis, which in fact depends essentially on the ability to dowse. It is commonly believed that this faculty is a special art, capable of being practised only by people who have some kind of psychic power. This is quite incorrect, for it is basically an exercise of the paranormal senses, which we all possess but which need to be educated. I am myself a reasonably down-to-earth individual, in no way psychic beyond having a firm conviction in the existence of higher levels of intelligence. It was thus with no great expectations that I began to experiment with dowsing, and was surprised to find that with practice I was able to develop a reasonable competence.

The faculty can, in fact, be cultivated much more readily than is generally assumed, though the development of a consistent ability requires patience and application. Major-General Scott-Elliot, President of the British Society of Dowsers, has said that from his experience with testing and helping people to learn the technique, only some 10 per cent were hopelessly insensitive. Of the remainder, a further 10 per cent showed exceptional promise, while 80 per cent could become reasonable dowsers if they wanted to, and found a useful outlet for their ability.

This last proviso, he maintained, was essential. No proper facility can be attained in a dilettante fashion. It is essential to have some sense of purpose if the education of the paranormal senses is to be successfully accomplished. In the present context the outlet is ready and waiting. It only remains to make a start, to which end a number of simple exercises can be undertaken. These are best discussed separately, and are set out in detail in appendix 1. If these are pursued with patience to attain an initial facility it is possible to obtain more advanced instruction from experts.

We have seen how the pendulum can answer qualitative questions involving a simple yes or no, but there are many instances where it is necessary to obtain an indication of degree or proportion—in other words, a quantitative assessment. This the pendulum can provide with precision, if it is asked to do so.

For this purpose it is convenient to use some form of rule or chart, on which the pendulum can indicate the extent of departure from the norm, or such other indication as may be required. For example, in the test on the nameplate previously mentioned, a chart could be prepared containing a series of radial lines at an angle of 20 degrees, numbered 0, 10, 20 . . . 90, 100. If the unknown material is placed over the origin of these lines, and the pendulum held over it, while the free hand is placed on a sample of copper to serve as a 'witness', the pendulum will swing over one of the radial lines indicating the actual percentage of copper in the sample; and the test can be repeated for other metals.

I once used such a chart to analyse a coin of unknown composition. It gave me 65 per cent copper and 25 per cent zinc, leaving 10 per cent unaccounted for. By trying a number of other metals as witnesses I found that the missing element was aluminium. But this again is by way of illustration, for without some knowledge of alloys I should not have been able to ask an intelligent question.

Other forms of chart can be used, suitable for specific types of investigation, and there is no need to discuss them in detail, though one particular form is mentioned in the appendix. They are, in fact, no more than a convenient means of focusing the attention of the dowser, and if properly used will provide a quantitative assessment of the relationship between any particular sample and an appropriate witness; and this can be used for much more subtle investigations than the simple examples so far quoted.

The essential conditions for the successful use of the pendulum are a quiet mind and clear and specific questioning. Without this, misleading answers will be obtained. It is not that the pendulum will not respond, but that the indications will be unreliable if the question is ambiguous. I once tested the suitability (for me) of some brown bread from which I confidently expected a positive response. To my surprise, the pendulum said no. But I had been testing it in its wrapping, and realized that I had been vaguely interrogating the whole package. By asking specifically 'Is this *bread* suitable?' I obtained a positive answer, and when I later tested the wrapping paper I found that it contained aluminium energy, to which I am allergic. Clearly this kind of vague questioning would be quite useless in the investigation of an obscure medical problem.

In a short introduction to dowsing issued by the Psionic Medical Society entitled *Simple Exercises with a Pendulum*, Carl Upton says:

> Before putting the pendulum into operation the dowser must have clearly in mind the question it is desired to elucidate. The question must be direct and be expressed in the simplest terms possible. Any ambiguity is bound to result in an ambiguous and inconclusive result. It is an axiom in dowsing that nonsense begets nonsense.
>
> When formulating a question to which an answer is required there must be no prejudice in the mind of the dowser. Any mental preconceptions or suggestions which occupy the mind of the operator are bound to confuse the dowsing faculty and the indications of the pendulum will be worthless. It is for this reason that 'arranged' tests to satisfy curiosity, to convince sceptics, or merely tricks and showmanship should be avoided at all costs. No serious dowser tolerates such impositions since anything outside of the pure and simple question with which the enquiry is concerned will nullify the findings and make the operation valueless and such superimposition is inevitable in the circumstances named.
>
> The history of dowsing is full of examples of this unintelligent misuse of the faculty, and the failures reflect not only the lack of knowledge and experience of the dowser but result in misunderstanding and often condemnation.

The pendulum, in fact, must not be used for trivialities. When first learning the technique it is permissible, in the quiet of one's own study or room, to make a variety of simple tests of no appreciable significance, in order to get the feel of the pendulum, and establish the pattern of its responses for oneself. But having acquired a consistent expertise, its use should be limited to matters of importance.

I remember a woman who was trying to demonstrate her prowess with this new toy saying 'Let us see whether my pussy has eaten her supper', which she could have verified quite simply by going to look for herself! It is essential to remember always that one is attempting to ask questions of an intelligent universe possessing a consciousness of a superior order. Any attempt to communicate with this higher level must be undertaken with a proper sense of scale.

Chapter 9

Medical Dowsing

We have discussed in broad terms the technique of using the pendulum, and it is not difficult to understand that with proper training and knowledge it is possible to interrogate a blood spot or other sample to obtain medical information. Any such investigation, of course, is not concerned with physical structure, but with the much more subtle energy content, and this can only be undertaken in an atmosphere of impersonal and fully educated inquiry.

This involves adequately informed and patient training. At the outset there is always the danger of subjective interpretations. In extreme cases questions may be based upon nothing but fantasy and the outcome can only be fantasy too. It is for this reason that it is standard practice in psionic medicine to use samples and witnesses derived usually from tissues and the *Materia Medica* used in homoeopathy. Such witnesses, used according to the techniques evolved, themselves pose the questions and the practitioner is minimally engaged. Indeed, the main use to which the mind of the practitioner is put in the process is to formulate the variety and sequence of witnesses to be employed in a particular case; and this formulation is necessarily based upon adequate knowledge and experience of clinical material. The only other function of the mental process is to interpret the results in terms of orthodox knowledge and nomenclature wherever possible; which again requires the necessary clinical experience.

The human mind is so conditioned by the influences to which it has been subjected over the centuries, and by contemporary education, prejudice and propaganda from all sides, that it is normally quite incapable of formulating questions untainted by this conditioning, and therefore intrinsically worthless.

In practice one sees many examples of users of a pendulum who become utterly enslaved by a mechnical addiction to this method of inquiry. Every aspect of their daily living becomes subject to 'pendulum censorship' and no move is made in any direction until the pendulum has issued its dictat in response to the futile stream of questions that emanate from the disturbed mind.

The only valid question is one posed by reality. Then a real answer may emerge. In the medical context, the reality in terms of the problems posed by diagnosis and treatment is the substantial 'witness' derived from living tissue; and, as has already been said, this by its very nature poses the valid question as soon as it is consciously related to other witnesses similarly derived. The practitioner's mind remains but a silent observer.

Extensive experience in psionic medicine leaves no doubt of the need to stress this point and bring to light the inherent dangers of use of the pendulum without recourse to valid knowledge and appropriate witnesses. The path of dowsing is strewn with increasing numbers of unfortunate people who have strayed into a cloud-cuckoo-land of fantasy and brought nothing but folly and worthless escapism into their lives; and if they have undertaken to help others, as they so often feel constrained to do by virtue of their own emptiness and need for self-justification, the results for their charges can be equally tragic.

It is for this reason that the Psionic Medical Society steadfastly refuses to publish detailed formulations of its techniques. These can only be communicated by personal instruction, which is available to qualified practitioners, and of which an increasing number are taking advantage.

It is therefore only possible to indicate in broad terms the practical basis of psionic analysis. Starting with an orthodox assessment of the patient's symptoms, and a knowledge of the case history, the practitioner will know from experience the possible miasmic or toxic influences which may be involved. A blood spot, or other sample, is then analysed with reference to appropriate witnesses of the suspected disorder, one or more of which indicate deviations from the norm, of greater or lesser severity. Again from experience, the practitioner will be aware of suitable (homoeopathic) remedies, and by touching with the free hand selected samples of such remedy, of different potencies, one or more may be found which restore the pendulum swing to normal, and this is prescribed accordingly.

It must be emphasized that this is no more than an illustration of the approach, for an actual analysis is much more detailed, including information as to the duration and frequency of the treatment. The essential point is that the indications obtained are precise and specific, and are related to the patient and not the symptoms.

The procedure usually adopted in psionic medicine can be divided into four stages, as follows:

1 The identification of inherited miasms resulting from acute infectious disease in parent or other forebear. This is followed by an assessment of the degree and distribution of the effects of the miasm or miasms throughout the systems, organs and tissues.

2 Identification of the toxic fall-out incurred as a result of acquired infectious illness or other dynamic causes in the individual concerned. A similar determination of degree and distribution is then made. When the diagnosis and analysis have been completed, an appropriate remedy must be selected psionically which is indicated as being able to neutralize the toxic emanations identified.

3 The effects on systemic and organic function in relation to the protoplasmic changes now effected must be assessed. All other aspects of the new situation both clinically and psionically must be taken into account. Residual gross toxaemia or tissue salt deficiency must be dealt with in the prescription of further remedies, if this is necessary. This is usually accomplished in stages, the most important systems being dealt with first; and not until complete functional balance at all levels is restored can a cure be claimed.

4 Attention may be given at this point to diet and other environmental factors, including psychological deviations which have not responded to the removal of the biological toxins. These may be adversely affecting the patient and offering a threat in the shape of further possible involvement in acute infectious disease.

Although emphasis has been laid on the purely medical approach to this work, the techniques are perfectly adaptable to dental, veterinary and other practice. Chronic and acute dental disorders arise from the same basic causes as those in any other part of the organism. The symptoms merely exhibit the form appropriate to the nature of the affected tissue. Psionic medicine offers the possibility of real preventive dental medicine because of its concern with predisposing causes and their elimination.

Another fruitful field, though as far as is known yet unexplored with psionic techniques, is soil and crop health. There is no reason to suppose that soil and crops under modern conditions of 'factory husbandry' have escaped their acute crises and toxic emanations establishing chronic disease states. With necessary research it should be possible to eliminate soil and crop miasms using psionic techniques and to restore good heart to the benefit of soil, plant, animal and man.

An aspect of medical dowsing which is of the utmost importance is the influence of faith. The intelligent practitioner, trained in skilled reasoning, will inevitably question whether unorthodox cures are not merely the result of credulity on the part of the patient—or even coincidence. There is, however, ample evidence that the results have a firmer basis. Not only is the existence of paranormal faculties scientifically established, but the records of psionic medical practice exhibit a consistent level of success.

Nevertheless, faith plays an important part in the process, not in the patient alone but in the mind of the practitioner. Faith is not the same as credulity, which is entirely subjective, but is the innate belief in a superior level, and it is noteworthy that animals and young children who have no knowledge of the fact that they are being treated are usually the best of patients; recovery is quick and uneventful.

As we grow up and become 'educated', this wordless acknowledgment of truth becomes atrophied. It is not merely that it is no longer adequately nourished, but that it is actively poisoned by the materialistic outlook, which cannot believe in anything beyond the interpretations of the senses. In such conditions the influences of the higher levels of reality not only find no soil in which to burgeon, but are entrapped and degraded by irrelevant detail.

This creates a considerable difficulty for the practitioner. It is not that a sceptical patient is *ipso facto* unable to be treated, but that the mental impartiality of the practitioner may be jeopardized. The place of faith, Upton suggests, in so far as it bears on the outcome of treatment, has its centre of gravity in the practitioner rather than the patient. It is a quality necessarily inherent in diagnosis and treatment—though it cannot substitute for poor technique or inadequate medical knowledge.

St Paul defined faith as 'The assurance of things hoped for, the evidence of things not seen.' This typifies the spirit in which the medical dowser approaches his task. He has stepped, as it were, into another dimension outside the region of the familiar—the region of clinical detail—into a realm in which the parts are integrated into a whole, but is unseen from the former standpoint; and it is from this state of unity that action emerges in terms of both diagnosis and treatment. Yet it is important to emphasize that he retains, but in its right place, the manifest evidence with which he was confronted by the afflicted patient.

There must be no division in the dowser's mind as he works. Disbelief in the patient's mind sows the seeds of division in the practitioner's, and the result is immediately in jeopardy. Naturally an experienced practitioner is able to retain impartiality and an adequate measure of freedom from most assaults, but not in every case; and he is wise to decline a case in which there is obvious disinclination to trust either diagnosis or treatment.

Experience has shown, further, that should there be scepticism and doubt in the mind of a third party closely associated with the patient this too can prejudice the outcome. It has been known, for example, for a sceptical doctor to refer a case for psionic medical diagnosis as a sort of test; perhaps even to discredit the technique. This scepticism conveys itself to the practitioner, either directly or through the patient, and unless he is able to preserve his integrity of mind, failure is usually inevitable. This, of course, is taken to discredit the system; but in reality the discredit reflects on the doctor.

Perhaps the most striking example of the effects of scepticism in the field of general dowsing has been demonstrated in popular television. Otherwise competent dowsers, known to be effective in their private capacity, have been rendered ineffective in the face of the television camera. Viewers in considerable numbers who watch these programmes do so essentially in a spirit of scepticism and doubt, even—such is human nature—a powerful wish to see the expert fail. The weight of such prejudice is immense and it is usually sufficient to render the dowser incapable of attaining that necessary freedom and innocence of mind to be able to function as he does when not under the stress of the forces of negation.

It therefore behoves every practitioner, experienced or tyro—and especially the latter—to avoid any occasion where there is likely to be a climate of disbelief. Psionic medicine requires of the practitioner a mind undisturbed by the clash of disputation—a state not easy to attain in the presence of those whose coin is dispute. Neither is it possible for such to take up the practice of psionic medicine and realize the potential it offers for themselves.

Chapter 10

The Basis of Psionic Medical Technique

It will be clear from the foregoing chapters that the pendulum, properly used, can provide valuable information about medical conditions which is not available to the orthodox approach. This information is utilized in psionic medical practice in a particular manner, having an established scientific basis, which must not be confused with the various usages popularly known as medical radiesthesia or radionics, which usually refer only to symptomatic states. The term 'psionic medicine' is specific, and may not be applied other than to the detailed procedure and principles evolved by Laurence and subsequently amplified by his colleagues.

Carl Upton has summarized the situation in the following terms. The techniques of psionic medicine, he says, involve on the one hand detailed knowledge and experience in the orthodox medical field, and on the other the ability to dowse in relation to samples and appropriate witnesses with the aid of suitable geometric patterns or rules to introduce the possibility of measurement in the evaluation of the results.

Essentially the technique requires the mental formulation of specific questions arising out of the known clinical data related to the patient's medical history and current complaints. To such questions the response to the trained practitioner comes in the form of reactions indicated by a hand-held pendulum which is used to measure deviations from the norm, by reference to an appropriate chart. A knowledge of anatomy, physiology, pathology, bacteriology and pharmacology and practical experience in these subjects is a basic requirement; in addition to which the principles of medicine and surgery and familiarity with the elements of psychology are needed to enable the practitioner to frame in his mind the necessary formulation to convey to the dowsing faculty. A set of co-ordinates, as it were, must first be established and this depends upon the experience of the practitioner. Then the dowsing faculty is enabled to respond in meaningful terms which can be understood in relation to the observed clinical data and history.

Whereas in orthodox medical diagnostic procedure use is made of inference and standardized references either in the intellectual memory or reference libraries, the logical conclusions being therefore indirect, in psionic medical techniques the conclusions reached are immediate and direct and stem from another dimension of knowledge.

Where, as in orthodox diagnostic procedures, standardized references are used it is not difficult to set down definite rules of procedure. But where individual sensitivity is involved as a means towards diagnosis it is not possible to represent this adequately in any text. Indeed, any attempt to do so could lead to many misleading notions and consequent distortions which could well prejudice the welfare of patient and reputation of practitioner. It is for this reason that the techniques of psionic medicine can only be taught verbally and in person by an experienced practitioner.

To enable any interested medical or dental practitioner to gain some familiarity in a preparatory way with the use of the pendulum some simple exercises appear in appendix 1. But the application of any facility thereby gained can only be related to the specific psionic medical techniques of diagnosis and remedy selection through personal instruction. It should perhaps be emphasized that until the candidate is able to use the pendulum successfully the techniques of psionic medicine cannot be taught. Equally a pendulist who does not have the necessary basic medical knowledge and experience cannot be taught either.

The systematic use of witnesses in the analysis has been established according to basic medical principles, and the witnesses themselves have, in a number of cases, been compounded as a result of the application of such principles. The same applies in remedy selection and the compounding of appropriate medication. This also conforms to the homoeopathic principle, which involves the use of the appropriate 'simillimum' at all stages of treatment, and the homoeopathic *Materia Medica* is freely used.

The well-known Bach remedies are also used on occasion. These affect the emotional aspects of the etheric body and are usually employed after the clearance of the miasmic imbalances.

An important feature of the method incorporates the use of

colour as an aid to diagnosis. Much has been written about the use of colour in certain forms of treatment but no reference is known to its use in specific diagnosis of causative factors in disease.

Laurence observed that infections reacted in a specific way to colours of the spectrum. He found that he could classify infectious diseases in terms of their colour relationships and he compiled a register of his findings. With this register he could immediately arrive at a conclusion as to the category into which the causative organism fell, either as a miasm or an acquired toxin. If a blood sample gave a reaction to a particular colour in the spectrum, then he knew that the patient concerned was affected by one of the organisms in the category indicated. This has proved to be an important aid to diagnosis since it eliminates the necessity for testing a large number of witnesses to determine the affecting organism.

Other methods have subsequently been adopted to facilitate the diagnostic and remedy selection procedures but the colour method still remains a most important aid. And from the point of view of research into the nature of the dynamic forces associated with micro-organic life the colour spectrum offers tremendous possibilities from which many conclusions about the nature of disease can be drawn—conclusions which are not apparent from morphological and other types of physical study.

Not only do the techniques provide diagnostic information of basic causes of imbalance in the vital dynamis and indicate the necessary remedies but they also indicate frequency and duration of medication. They are also used to show the effects of other forms of medication in terms of their influence on the vital constitution and can thus prevent the occurrence of possible side effects that might result from the administration of unsuitable allopathic drugs.

It was stated earlier that psionic medicine adds a further dimension to the medical art; and this can be appreciated by considering the three aspects of creation found in ancient cosmologies, as they relate to the organization of living physical matter. There is first the attribute of idea or form—the unmanifest pattern of everything that exists. The second attribute is substance, which gives material expression to the pattern; and finally there is the reconciling attribute of life, the carrier of the dynamic potential which sustains the triad.

There is a significant correlation here. The affirmation of the creative purpose—which essentially involves health or wholeness—relates to the first attribute, involving treatment of the underlying patterns. Allopathy, in its concern with physical symptoms and body chemistry, is related to the material attribute. Psionic medicine and homoeopathy are concerned with the vital animating forces. They have, as it were, a foot in both worlds and hold the key to reconciliation.

This is possible by the use of the paranormal sensitivity which, in one of its manifestations, appears as the dowsing faculty. This is not employed to analyse symptoms, or chains of logical cause and effect, but seeks to discover the fundamental disharmonies which give rise to the clinical disturbances.

These three aspects are illustrated by the latest developments in molecular biology. Research has shown a fundamental connection between the amino acids, which comprise the protein molecule, and the constituent of the genes called DNA, acting through an intermediary substance RNA.

Biologists ascribe to DNA the function of the carrier of genetic information. Protein is the principal material of which the tissues of the body are made and RNA is the catalyst that unites the two into a living whole. Hence in terms of the creative triad, it would seem that DNA provides the expression of the form, protein gives substance to the genetic pattern, while RNA is the vehicle of the life attribute.

The techniques of psionic medicine involve the use of witnesses which are brought into dowsing relationship with a specimen—usually of blood, hair or saliva—of the patient under examination. If witnesses derived from DNA, RNA and the amino acids are used, these can immediately give valuable information concerning the three fundamental attributes of the organism: genetic, dynamic and biochemical. Qualitative imbalances in any of these components of the total life of the organism can be detected and evaluated with the help of further witnesses and appropriate measuring scales.

Psionic medicine stresses the necessity to establish at the outset the basic cause of symptoms before treatment is started. It now becomes clearer that information at genetic level is the first requirement, for it is here that the pattern is established which will influence physical structure, producing abnormalities as a state of disease. This is the level at which consideration must be given to inherited miasms which derive from the experience of disease in forebears, the commonest of which are the miasms of tuberculosis, syphilis and the sycotic group. This is the point where many of the chronic symptoms of disease in the individual are initiated, irrespective of environment. This is the blueprint stage, the determinant of the form of the organic structure of which protein is ultimately the major constituent. The appropriate witness is DNA. With information gained from psionic analysis and with homoeopathic potencies of the correct dynamic order, miasmic disturbances of genetic patterns may be corrected.

It is perhaps necessary to point out here that the symptoms that occur as a result of a particular miasm usually bear no relation to those associated with the original disease in the forebear which gave rise to the miasm genetically. For example, the tubercular miasm can account for the most diverse range of symptoms, including those of asthma, eczema, migraine, diabetes, dental caries, Hodgkin's disease and many other so-called incurable diseases involving various organs and systems.

Qualitative changes influencing the building and maintenance processes that constantly go on in the cells are associated with the vital forces. The appropriate witness is RNA. These changes often occur following acute infections or after the use of their derivatives used in immunization. They are known in psionic medicine as acquired toxins, and again predispose to symptoms apparently unrelated to the infection. They are removed homoeopathically.

As was explained in chapter 5 the acquired toxins may make an impression upon the genetic pattern and establish a chronic predisposition similar to that occurring in inherited miasms. It may be through some such mechanism that the miasmic chain is established. In practice it is found that these acquired toxins may sometimes appear when DNA is used as a witness, especially if all miasms have been removed previously.

Protein, and associated substances, taken from the environment in the form of food, provides the material basis—the second attribute. Deficiencies or inferior quality are reflected in the cell substance and may precipitate symptoms. They may also affect vitality. The state of the physical organs and the conditions of the environment play an important part at this level. The witness used is taken from the amino acids, and their concomitants.

To understand the psionic medical approach it is necessary to extend one's thinking beyond the ideas of conventional acceptance; but this does not mean that psionic medicine is a mere theory. On the contrary it is of the greatest practical value, once its techniques have been mastered, as is proved by its record of successes, some of which are detailed in chapter 13.

As has been repeatedly emphasized, the analysis and treatment is essentially individual, not relying on standardized diagnosis and treatment; nor does it involve animal experimentation. There is today much interest in transplant and 'spare part' surgery. But such techniques, with their moral issues and considerable expenditure of manpower and resources, might well be avoided by psionic analysis earlier in life, before irreversible damage has occurred.

Similarly, mental illness could be reduced extensively. It is Laurence's experience that a large percentage of cases in this category are due to inherited miasms and acquired toxins; possibly aggravated by external conditions, including modern drugs, but not necessarily caused by them primarily.

Moreover, psionic techniques can be used to test the effect of conventional synthetic drugs on the individual vitality. They also provide a means of checking intolerance and sensitivity to aluminium, fluorine, mercury, radiation and other toxic factors with which the individual may come into contact; and if these are present, they may be neutralized.

If some of the resources at present squandered on the attempted amelioration of physical symptoms could be diverted to the study of the dynamic causes of illness, new horizons would appear in medical research which could lead to a more comprehensive health service.

Chapter 11

Causative Factors in Illness

One of the principal advantages of psionic medicine is its ability to treat not only acute conditions, but chronic states, even those which are normally regarded as incurable. This possibility has already been discussed in the preceding chapters, but it will be helpful to consider it in more specific terms.

To this end we cannot do better than refer to an article by Carl Upton, 'Acute infectious and chronic disease' (*Journal of the Psionic Medical Society*, vol. 1, no. 5).

From the point of view of health or wholeness, he says, it is difficult to draw a dividing line between acute and chronic illness. Both indicate a loss of equilibrium in the vital energies which maintain the integrity and normal functional activity of the organism. But in contemporary medical practice such a division is usually accepted, probably in the first place because of the differences in physical symptoms recognized and secondly because of the limitations imposed by techniques of diagnosis.

The importance of finding possible relationships between acute and chronic disease lies in the fact that it could lead to a deeper understanding of causation. The seeds of a chronic 'incurable' degenerative illness could lie in some acute infection suffered perhaps in childhood or, in the light of Hahnemann's concept of miasms, in an acute infectious disease in a forebear.

Modern medical textbooks list a great number of diseases, each bearing an appropriate label. But a seeker after health would find little or no help, indeed would perhaps find greater confusion from such a classification, because of the lack of evidence of meaningful bridges between the entities described.

It is doubtful, for example, if the reader would find a reference to a link between, say, tubercular infection in a grandfather and chronic migraine, diabetes, asthma, eczema or dental caries in grandchildren. Yet, if the organism (which includes essential inherited characteristics) is regarded as a whole, such a possibility cannot be ruled out. The question might equally well be asked: What is the possibility of a connection between measles or a streptococcus infection, malaria or vaccinosis, with chronic diseases which might involve symptoms in cardio-vascular, genito-urinary, digestive, nervous or other vital systems? Or even with cancer?

The crux of the matter seems to lie in the approach. If one draws conclusions only from changes observed in structure of tissues or cells or in molecular composition, these conclusions are only valid in terms of the physical characteristics of molecule or cell. They can have no reference to the vital dynamic formative forces in which we live, move and have our being. If these conclusions are then applied in diagnosis, causation is only seen in terms of structural change or effect.

On the other hand if one could find a way to gain direct knowledge of the forces involved in organic life, then the structural changes observed would become understandable in relation to a context far transcending that of physical form alone. Temporal and spatial dimensions could be bridged and causative relationships of a new order be established. The medical textbooks could be rewritten.

The physical symptoms associated with the disease called diabetes, for example, may be clinically observed. These symptoms are known usually to be accompanied by certain changes of structure in the cells of the pancreatic gland. The conclusion is drawn therefore that diabetes is caused by physical changes in the pancreas.

A study, however, of the formative energies related to the function and development of the gland may indicate a dynamic constitutional imbalance which is leading to structural and functional weakness or stress. Further investigation may show that this imbalance in the vital forces is associated with inherited tendencies derived from parent or grandparent; perhaps even having its origin in a serious infectious disease such as tuberculosis in the relative concerned. Here then, one may be much nearer the mark in stating the cause of the disease.

Incidentally, once the symptoms of diabetes occur and degeneration in the cell structure of the pancreas has taken place, it is usually accepted that no cure is possible because the physical changes are irreversible. The cause, in other words, from the purely structural point of view, cannot be removed. However, if imbalance in the vital energies is observed early enough, it can be corrected. Moreover, if physical degeneration is only present to a limited degree, the symptoms of diabetes will not develop further if the basic cause has been removed.

By the use of psionic techniques it is possible to study these dynamic formative energies, and thereby to obtain answers to many questions that arise out of the physical behaviour of the organism. The faculty may be applied to elucidate many of the complexities of the metabolic processes, both in health and disease; and such information, allied to a discriminative knowledge derived from experience gained in clinical medicine and surgery, can disclose the basic causes of disease.

Disturbances of vital balance can be detected which frequently appear as a persistent factor, or common denominator linking acute and chronic symptoms, both in the individual and in the family. Over a period of time a consistent inhibition of the vital energy may produce a condition of disharmony which can result in a variety of symptomatic structural changes in the body, apparently unrelated to one another physically, but which all stem from the same derangement of the vital energy.

When a state of dynamic balance is restored, the various symptoms and diseases may disappear with no further intervention, proving that the cause of the disorders lay not in tissue structure and physical composition, but in the natural energy patterns characteristic of the individual concerned. Laurence's experience has provided a wealth of evidence in support of this. He has evolved a precise system of detection, identification and measurement of energy imbalances affecting cells, tissues, organs and systems; and has been able to study the effect of homoeopathic medication on these energy patterns resulting in the amelioration of the clinical symptoms.

The dividing lines between acute infectious and chronic disease have, for him, largely disappeared and he is thus able to arrive at basic diagnoses embracing, in a large number of cases, causative factors extending sometimes far back in the line of inheritance. Armed with this knowledge, chronic 'incurable' degenerative disease ceases in most cases to present the insoluble problems it does to medical systems based only upon observations of physical structure and chemistry.

The work of Hahnemann in homoeopathy, and more recently that of Laurence in psionic medicine, appears to indicate that accompanying the gross pathological and bacteriological changes associated with acute infectious disease there is also a subtle emanation, and this emanation is characteristic of the type of infection. In other words, there may be a tubercular emanation or a measles emanation, quite distinct from the clinical infections of tuberculosis or measles. The presence of this emanation is not detected by standard diagnostic techniques since they are limited to chemico-physical investigation.

This 'fall-out' (which Hahnemann called a miasm) persists as an active biological toxic factor after the macroscopic and microscopic symptoms have resolved and the infection is apparently cured. It produces basic functional changes in the protoplasm which in turn can lead to multiplicity of chronic symptoms, the cause of which is unrecognized except by psionic techniques. There is reason to suppose also that the period of persistence of activity or 'life' of a miasm, as well as its depth of penetration, is characteristic for each infection. Some have a longer period of activity and a more profound impact than others. Indeed, in some cases, tuberculosis for example, the toxic energies may be genetically reflected through subsequent generations of offspring. This can bring aberrations of structure which can perpetuate the pathological situation in the family, though in other forms than those generally accredited to a tubercular infection.

It seems that most chronic and degenerative states of disease and symptoms may stem from this subtle cause. And this would account for the fact that they do not respond, in the curative sense, to allopathic symptomatic treatment. To be successful, treatment must be capable of neutralizing the toxic energies concerned and this calls for subtle remedies such as those provided by homoeopathic potencies.

Acute infection is generally believed to occur as a result of an infiltration of pathogenic or disease-producing micro-organisms. These attack the tissues and multiply and bring about a situation in which germs, their waste products, the results of tissue destruction, and the cells of the body delegated to resist the infection all assemble locally or spread throughout the body to produce the crisis called acute infectious disease.

But if a deeper understanding is to be had, then a consideration of the process from the point of view of a number of other factors, including that of the vital energies, must be undertaken. For example, one must consider polarity in micro-organic life. It has long been recognized that certain micro-organisms associated with the body may exhibit two roles. They may be present as saphrophytes or pathogens. That is, they may be harmless and even helpful to the normal organic processes or they may attack the tissues and cause symptoms of acute infection. We must inquire why this change of polarity occurs. Why, for example, can a staphylococcus aureus germ or a bacillus coli be found in healthy tissues in perfectly normal function at one time and yet at another obviously rampant in the cause of acute infection?

A good deal of research is necessary into this most important aspect since it involves a link in the chain that ultimately appears to lead to chronic disease.

And again, why epidemics? Undoubtedly many forms of energy disturbance, both environmental and constitutional, could be the cause of a change of polarity. There is evidence that points to the fact, for instance, that hyperfunction of the adrenal medulla, with the over-secretion of adrenalin, may be capable of changing polarity. This is possibly a common factor in a stress society. Again, the indiscriminate and repetitive use of antibiotics may bring about a situation in which polarity changes take place. And this polarity change, clearly demonstrated in psionic medicine, is the first step on the road to some form of chronic illness.

Cosmic factors, planetary influences, season, climate, geography, food and a host of other environmental forces all play a part in the predisposition to acute infection, epidemic or otherwise. Psychological factors also play a part without doubt, together with the influences of social, economic and other circumstances. And, as such, they may form the conditions in which, through the incidence of infection, in many cases the stage is set for a disturbance of the vital constitutional energies, leading to chronic illness in one form or another either in the individual or in future generations.

There is little doubt that, once chronic disease is established, the vital resources necessary to the maintenance of constitutional balance in the face of adverse environmental factors are diminished; and so it is that the elimination of miasms and acquired toxins resulting from past infections should be given priority, not only from the point of view of the removal of the chronic symptoms wherever possible but as a measure limiting the incidence of acute infectious illness in the future.

The practice of homoeopathy can claim a considerable record of success in chronic and inherited conditions because its remedies have the necessary dynamic potency to neutralize the toxic biological emanations concerned. It can also take credit for success in acute conditions and in prevention. Its weakness, however, lies in the fact that the means used to determine the precise nature of the miasms and acquired toxins are subject to a wide margin of error. Prescription is also imprecise. With the introduction of the techniques of psionic medicine by Laurence this margin of error has been considerably reduced, and an experienced diagnostician should have no difficulty either in identifying causes or in selecting appropriate homoeopathic potencies.

Psionic medicine, which depends on the psionic faculty as the means capable of perceiving and identifying toxic biological energies, has opened up the possibility of a far more comprehensive diagnosis and therapy than is available in any other system of medicine. It has confirmed the Unitary Theory of Disease propounded by McDonagh. The miasms or acquired toxic emanations from a state of acute disease are active forces which invite involvement since nature always tends towards restoration of balance. This enveloping reaction occurs in the basic protoplasm which then exists in an over-contracted state. And it is this aberration in the structure which gives rise to the multiplicity of symptoms that are possible. With the neutralizing of the harmful toxic energies the protoplasm takes on its normal density. This is accompanied by a release of vital energies formerly held in check and fully vitalized health becomes possible provided no irreversible damage has occurred prior to treatment, when all that can be expected is an arrest of the degenerative processes caused by the toxic biological fall-out.

Chapter 12

The Psionic Method in Dental Medicine

The discussions so far have been concerned with the broad aspects of disease, but a by no means inconsiderable part of medical practice is concerned with dental hygiene in which psionic techniques afford normally unsuspected possibilities. There are two attitudes towards the problem of dental disorders, the preventative and the conservative, both of which are applied in their appropriate context.

The conditions of contemporary society inevitably throw the emphasis on the techniques of conservation. The dental surgeon is faced with immediate and pressing demands for the salvage of teeth which have already been attacked by disease, often irremediably; in the course of which new techniques of pain relief and mechanical restoration are evolved, with an expanding array of materials and equipment.

It would be fair to say, however, that the average practitioner regards salvage as the least satisfactory aspect of his skill and endeavours to apply his knowledge to prevention. There are here two schools of thought. One believes that dental disorders are largely the fault of the environment, so that although restorative surgery has a certain preventive value in ensuring adequate masticatory functioning (and aesthetic satisfaction) it must be reinforced by good oral hygiene, and proper stimulation of the dental supporting tissues.

In this category is the controversial subject of fluoridation of public water supplies. It has been claimed that the application of trace concentrations of fluorine preparations to the teeth prevents dental caries. Scientific evidence is divided concerning these claims and many regard them as non-proven or even potentially dangerous.

Apart from these localized measures, however, there is the aspect of diet and nutrition. The environmentalists consider that here lies the key—or at least a major portion of it—to unlock the door to health and ensure prevention of disease, dental or otherwise. A great deal has been said and written on this subject, from the simple advice to avoid excesses, or to cut out refined carbohydrates and other processed and chemically contaminated foods, or to adopt vegetarian habits.

It is argued, with justification, that the ways of life of contemporary society in industrialized communities are not likely to produce an environment in which a state of health can flourish. Even the physical activity necessary to healthy metabolic exchange is at a premium in a world in which mechanical transport and mechanical aids in general usurp almost all normal human functions.

In the face of these conditions one must surely look elsewhere for solutions. This is the view of the alternative school which seeks a deeper understanding of the background to the distressingly prevalent troubles. Dental disorders are seen as merely specific and localized departures from overall health, so that the problem resolves itself into the location of the underlying causes of such departure, and the discovery of means whereby it may be prevented or at least ameliorated.

It is here that psionic methods are invaluable, and once again we can quote Carl Upton, whose training and subsequent experience as a salvage dentist did not satisfy his intuitive belief in the need to study the causes of the disorders, to which he found the key in the work of George Laurence. In a paper entitled 'The psionic method in preventive dental medicine', published by the Psionic Medical Society, he says:

> Laurence, with his extensive knowledge of clinical morbid anatomy, physiology and pathology, combined with the experience derived from his researches into what he refers to as the 'formative forces' has been able to establish definite causal relationships between disturbances produced in the formative body by certain diseases or infections, and clinical symptoms, usually of chronic disease, in the physical body.
>
> Under the influence of a scientific outlook devoted solely to a consideration of the structure of matter and its behaviour, medical and dental practice is conditioned to observe and

treat the physico-chemical organism within the limits of the technical knowledge in which it has been educated. Since knowledge of the vital dynamic forces involved in nature does not fall within these limits, medicine and dentistry have been deprived, other than in the case of a real intuitive clinical sense developed through long experience, of the opportunity to come to grips with and understand the deep inherent causes of disease which lie in the vital being of man.

Whereas observation of the physical personality can be carried out with the aid of the five senses and with the assistance of laboratory techniques and instruments, that of the vital force determining the nature of the individual can only be achieved through the use of a different range of senses, involving the exercise of the psionic faculty.

Every doctor and dentist knows that the influences involved in heredity play a fundamental part in the make-up of their patient's constitution. They do not necessarily know the character of these influences. They are not thus aware of the nature of the unsuspected causes of ill-health that stem from the chain of inheritance; unless they have turned their attention in the direction indicated by Hahnemann and Laurence.

To understand dental disease it is necessary to examine not only the relationship between the person and his environment and the character of that environment, but also to probe the relationship between the physical person and his vital essence. If this can be done then dental practice takes on a very different meaning—a new dimension is added.

Although the immediate salvage necessity may remain, including modifications to the environment wherever desirable and possible, parallel with this, treatment can be instituted with a view to the correction of inherent causes which are giving rise to a weakness in the structure and to faulty metabolism of the dental tissues.

Laurence has shown that not only the influences of serious disease in a forebear can disturb the balance of the vital force field of later generations, expressing as miasms, but that certain infectious diseases have their immediate effect in producing what he refers to as 'hangovers' or acquired dynamic toxins in the formative body. Both constitute causative factors which must be eliminated before cure in the real sense of the word is possible. From the dental point of view, however meticulous the salvage operations or care in choice of food and way of life, the patient remains constantly at risk of dental lesions while miasms and dynamic toxins remain unresolved.

Over an increasing number of cases diagnosed and treated by the psionic method where dental disorders occur, the high, almost universal, incidence of the tubercular miasms is noted. Although both human and bovine miasms are frequently present, there is evidence, not yet fully confirmed, that the miasms of bovine tuberculosis are especially significant as a possible predisposition to dental caries.

Both the miasms and the acquired dynamic toxin associated with measles infection also occur very frequently. Less frequent are the miasms of syphilis and gonorrhoea. Among the acquired dynamic toxins regularly encountered are those associated with staphylococcus aureus, streptococcus, bacillus coli and bacillus coli Gaertner, bacillus Morgan, bacillus Proteus, bacillus catarrhalis, poliomyelitis and the toxins related to vaccination and aluminium. It is not yet confirmed that all of these have any direct bearing on dental disorders, although without doubt the bacillus coli and the vaccinosis toxins are significant in predisposing to paradontal conditions.

It is considered of great importance, now we have the techniques of psionic medicine, that the diagnosis and elimination of miasms and acquired toxins in children should be carried out wherever possible and on an increasing scale as trained operators become available. Not only do children respond so readily and so effectively to this treatment but, what is of far reaching benefit, the chain of miasms is broken. Children so treated are no longer 'carriers' of inimical influences and thus ensure for their own children a better expectancy of health from the outset. During adolescence and child-bearing years any acquired dynamic toxins arising from acute infections or other causes should be eliminated. Deficiency of any of the active elements of vitamins or essential minerals, which often accompanies a disturbance in the vital force field, requires to be made good.

It is evident from these remarks that psionic techniques provide valuable assistance in combating the modern scourge of debilitating dental disease. This arises from the introduction of a new dimension into the therapy, as may be illustrated clinically from practical experience in relation to dental caries.

In the narrowest sense, the clinical picture presented by this disease is a breakdown in the hard dental tissues. Mechanical techniques are used to remove diseased tissues and provide substitute functional restorations. This is the main field in which the dental surgeon works, but the scope of his inquiry is widened by consideration of environmental factors. Poor local hygiene and dietetic imbalance are known to play a role in the production of tissue breakdown, so that in addition to mechanical restoration increasing attention is being given to preventive measures.

Such measures, however, are still concerned with physical causation, whereas psionic techniques introduce a different dimension of diagnosis and treatment. In a large number of cases showing the incidence of dental caries psionic medical analysis has demonstrated the presence of inherited miasms. These are usually of the tubercular, particularly the bovine, group as already mentioned. In other words there is a genetic predisposition to the disease of dental caries. This of course may have been long suspected by dental clinicians but the nature and cause of the predisposition has not been apparent from work in the purely physical aspects of diagnosis and therapy. It has required the introduction of the new dimension opened up by psionic medical techniques to arrive at an understanding of basic factors involved in the causation of the disease and the means for its eradication.

Whereas dental surgical techniques and environmental preventive measures have succeeded in raising the level of dental functional efficiency to a certain point they have not been able to reduce the incidence of the disease from the genetic standpoint. This now becomes possible through psionic diagnosis and the removal of the causative miasms concerned.

For the dental surgeon who wishes to add this new dimension to his practice, the basic necessities are a knowledge of the homoeopathic *Materia Medica* and an ability to employ the psionic faculty, both of which require a period of training. But with such equipment the treatment can be of a far more comprehensive and deeper nature, taking into account the whole man, with which one is fundamentally concerned in the pursuit of health.

Chapter 13

Psionic Medicine in Practice

It has already been explained that there is no standardized routine in psionic diagnosis and medication. The treatment is, and must be, entirely individual. There is often more than one underlying cause, each of which requires attention in order of its relative importance, and the condition of the patient must be continually monitored. Moreover, the initial steps to correct a vital imbalance can sometimes produce tissue reactions associated with the detoxication—a well-known effect known as homoeopathic aggravation; and it is frequently found that after detoxication is completed a kind of nucleic depletion develops, resulting in what is called the negative phase, which requires appropriate treatment.

The trained practitioner is well aware of these effects, which do not arise from incorrect diagnosis, but are part of the normal operation of the *Vis Medicatrix Naturae* and are allowed for accordingly. They are mentioned here to emphasize once again that the effective use of psionic medical techniques can only be attained by adequate training and experience, allied to a thorough knowledge of medical principles. Given these conditions, however, psionic medicine has been proved to cure a wide variety of disorders which have not responded to orthodox treatment, and it will be useful to cite, by way of illustration, some practical examples.

To this end we can select from the journals of the Psionic Medical Society a number of representative case histories. To be of value, however, these must be quoted in detail, which would introduce a certain distraction in the narrative. Hence it will be simpler to indicate here a variety of disorders which have responded successfully to psionic treatment, and to include the details of typical cases in an appendix to which reference may be made as appropriate (Appendix 3).

A widespread complaint today is migraine, in which the patient suffers blinding headaches accompanied by other distressing symptoms for no apparent cause. In its severe form it is a prostrating malady whose victims may suffer recurring attacks which disrupt their work and happiness. Orthodox medical research has indicated a certain pattern in the symptoms, and has devised palliative treatments; but the prolonged use of these remedies, such as ergotamine, is accompanied by debilitating side effects, and the basic causes remain elusive. Psionic analysis has established that the effects are the result of miasmic disturbances, either hereditary or acquired, and that by appropriate treatment the malady can be permanently cured.

Relatively mild cases are usually found to arise from unsuspected acquired toxins. One example is a lady who had suffered from recurring headaches which at the age of 43 were becoming intolerable. Psionic analysis disclosed a malaria toxin, a hangover from an attack in her childhood. Removal of this toxin effected a complete cure.

A second case was that of an ex-RAF officer who experienced severe headaches following minor ailments such as intestinal infections. This was found to be the result of malaria and dysentery toxins, the removal of which cleared the trouble.

The majority of cases, however, are due to inherited miasms, often reinforced by acquired infections such as measles. Typical examples are as follows:

Case 1 Mr C.W., aged 57

The onset of migraine, with severe headaches, nausea and vomiting, occurred at approximately 18 years of age.

Attacks, which were often associated with events in which an element of emotional strain was involved, usually lasted for some hours and responded to light sedation and sleep. With advancing years the duration of the attacks increased until the usual pattern was extended over three days, often commencing on awakening in the morning.

For some years the attacks appeared to be linked in some sort of rhythmic pattern, often occurring at weekends. Certain foods were thought to increase susceptibility. The disrupting effect of the disease drove the patient to seek all forms of treatment in an attempt to get relief. Orthodox medication with ergotamine tartrate and other drugs failed to bring results, and resort had to be made to strong sedatives containing codeine, plus attempts to remain quiet in a darkened room.

In 1966 a psionic medical diagnosis was undertaken which disclosed the existence of tubercular miasms of both strains—Bovine and Koch. Treatment was commenced and continued over a period of several weeks. Since that time there has been no recurrence of the characteristic attacks. Occasional headaches, following periods of stress, have occurred but have responded immediately to mild sedation.

A number of further cases are listed in appendix 3 which provide further illustration of the true causes of this malady.

Another distressing complaint, particularly prevalent in children, is asthma, often accompanied by eczema. There is a very extensive record of the successful treatment of such cases by psionic methods. This ailment often requires prolonged homoeopathic medication since the causes may be multiple and deep-seated, but with patience a complete cure can be effected.

A typical example is as below:

Case 2 F.A., female aged 42

Acute and debilitating asthmatic attacks, which failed to respond to orthodox medical treatment and became progressively worse, brought this patient to the point of desperation. When first seen she was in considerable distress and required constant attention. Breathing was extremely difficult and even between attacks there was great difficulty in getting breath. There was a bad medical history, some of which was associated with a spell in the tropics. Brucellosis, aspergillosis, hookworm and pneumonia were all mentioned; and a persistent cough was accompanying the other symptoms.

A psionic analysis showed tubercular miasms of both TB and TK forms. There was also an indication of meningeal involvement and the brucellosis toxin.

A single dose of Bacillinum, followed by typical treatment for the miasms and the toxins lasting about two months, brought a most gratifying response, all symptoms being cleared and the patient becoming free from the asthma and breathlessness.

Interesting in this case was the dramatic response that occurred after the initial single dose of homoeopathic medicine. There was virtually a complete cessation of the distressing symptoms and no further inhalations or allopathic medicines were necessary.

About a year later the patient caught a cold and this resulted in a rather persistent cough which lasted for some weeks, but which responded to the appropriate homoeopathic medicine directed to the removal of the 'hangover' from the cold toxins.

Now, some three years later, the patient remains well and free from symptoms.

Perhaps even more distressing are cases of asthma in young children, and here psionic treatment can save untold misery, as is exemplified in the following case:

Case 3 B.M., male, aged 3½

This child developed asthma and eczema in the first year of his life. He went, in his mother's words, 'from one attack to another and I was in despair'.

In April 1969 a psionic diagnosis was done, which showed a double miasm of TK/TB together with a 'hangover' of vaccinia. Treatment was started, and by November his mother reported that in spite of a cold he had had practically no return of the asthma; after that he continued to improve until his mother now states she feels he is completely cured. She writes in April 1970, 'As a widow, this treatment of my son has completely changed my life. Before, I was afraid to leave him, due to the severity of the attacks. Now he is a happy contented child, whereas before he was a silent little wraith. I bless the day this knowledge [of psionic treatment] first came to hand.'

These are but two examples of the successful treatment of a malady which manifests itself in a variety of unpleasant ways. A number of further cases are quoted in the appendix, which illustrate the essentially individual approach of psionic techniques in the location and treatment of the underlying causes.

Psionic medicine is by no means confined to the treatment of the more common recalcitrant ailments. A disease which is causing some concern today is brucellosis (undulant fever) of which several cases are quoted in the appendix, which also includes case histories of a variety of chronic illnesses such as Hodgkin's disease, coeliac disease, liver disorders and so forth, often regarded as incurable but which respond to psionic medical treatment.

In addition there are records of the successful treatment of psychological disturbances such as schizophrenia and mental disorders. A particular example of this was the following:

Case 4 Mrs X., aged 73. Hypochondria

For thirty years this patient had been under various treatments for general ill-health and depression, finding life an increasing burden and weariness as she got older. She complained of chronic flatulence, constipation, no desire to eat, nausea, an inability to relax and no energy.

She had had a great deal of psychological and psychiatric treatment. ECT had been tried with no result except an increase in her loss of memory. She was finally categorized as a chronic hypochondriac for whom nothing could be done.

At this point she came reluctantly under psionic medical treatment with no hope and indeed with a very negative and unco-operative attitude. A psionic analysis showed the presence of an hereditary syphilitic miasm together with an intestinal toxaemia due to b. Morgan. This combination was affecting her adrenals, thyroid and portal system and the central and autonomic nervous systems. The indicated remedy was a single dose of high potency RNA (Nx). This eliminated the miasmic condition, and from this point, with many ups and downs, she gradually regained her mental and physical health and lost all the symptoms which had plagued her for so many years.

Appropriate treatment was continued for another ten months, as such cases are very liable to pick up or develop an intercurrent infection such as a staph. aur. or an atypical b.coli, as in fact she did. Continuing treatment was thus needed to deal with the temporary loss of dynamic balance, but she finally reported that she felt very fit, with a good appetite and plenty of energy; and that it was wonderful to feel so well.

This case, together with others of a similar nature, throws new light on the increasingly prevalent mental and psychological disorders which defy orthodox treatment. The ability to detect and remedy the underlying miasmic disturbances by psionic methods affords real hope for sufferers from these conditions.

Experience in fact is providing overwhelming confirmation of McDonagh's contention that there is only one basic disease, which arises from imbalance of the protein. This manifests itself in a bewildering variety of symptoms, some of miasmic origin, others due to acquired toxins including the usually unsuspected influence of aluminium energies. A selection of detailed case histories will be found in appendix 3.

We can conveniently conclude this chapter with an extract from 'Psionic medicine in general practice', *Journal of the Psionic Medical Society* (vol. 1 no. 3), by Dr John Porterfield, MA, MB, BChir (Cantab) who reinforced his orthodox knowledge by the appropriate training in psionic techniques, and makes the following observations:

> The idea that toxins remain in the body after a disease has apparently been cured was puzzling at first until I thought about rheumatic fever. This is a disease which may occur after a streptococcal sore throat. The acute manifestations pass off in a few weeks, but the after-effects may continue in the body undetected by laboratory investigation until they come out in chronic kidney, heart or joint disease after an interval of years. The current orthodox explanation for this is that it is an auto-immune reaction which is initiated by the toxin of the streptococcus. This fits in very well with the concept of toxins as hangovers from past infections. Such toxins clearly exist, though as yet they cannot be found by orthodox techniques, and it is reasonable to consider that others which are dowsed in psionic medicine, but which are unknown to conventional medicine, e.g. measles and aluminium toxins, may also exist.
>
> Inherited miasms or toxins are a real stumbling block to the orthodox, and yet they are only a specific explanation of what is described in every textbook as being 'hereditary'. We know that human constitutions differ, that some families are prone to migraine, or to diabetes, or that individual members of a family may have poor physical or mental health throughout life. The laboratory has been unable to detect any inherited toxins by such methods as antibody titres, so the conventional scientist accepts that the cause of inherited conditions lies in the genes, although he cannot prove this. The psionic

practitioner also says that the cause of inherited conditions lies in the genes, but that it is on a non-material level, detectable at present only by the supersensory techniques of dowsing, and he is able to identify the inherited toxins responsible for disease.

Another concept which was new to me was the role in disease of the bacterial flora of the gut. In the healthy, emotionally balanced man the normal bacterial inhabitant of the bowel is the bacillus coli. This is non-toxic to man. When a man is under some emotional strain there is a corresponding subtle change throughout his organism and in this new environment of tension the bacillus coli is unable to flourish. A mutant strain tends to replace it, but the newcomer produces a toxin which poisons the system of the host resulting in symptoms of indigestion, malaise, headache, skin eruption and so on. This concept, which has in fact been demonstrated by Dr Paterson in Glasgow, helps to explain the relationship between emotion and the diseases of stress which the general practitioner sees daily in the surgery.

Even in the early stages of learning these psionic techniques the practitioner develops a change of attitude to illness. The textbook summing up of many diseases—'cause unknown', 'hereditary', 'constitutional', 'palliative treatment only'—all this loses its meaning. Disease becomes a challenge which may be answerable. Patients with chronic disease who come up to the surgery month after month for a repeat of tablets, either a bit better, or a bit worse, become interesting. Why do they have their diseases? The general practitioner with appropriate training has the means of diagnosis and treatment at his fingertips through the exercise of psionic techniques.

Chapter 14

The Whole Man

It will be evident from the foregoing chapters that psionic medicine is an essentially practical system. At the same time it is equally evident that it is not just a new variety of fringe medicine, but is based on the acknowledgment of superior levels of Intelligence which are responsible for all the manifestations of the phenomenal world; and it is the intuitive faith in this superior level which has inspired the new dimensions of understanding which have been emerging in recent times.

The growing recognition of this need for a more comprehensive understanding prompted Professors Alberto Lodispoto and Andrea Salvati of the Medical Faculty of the University of Rome to convene in May 1973 the first World Congress of l'Altra Medicina. This was held in San Remo with the object of finding a common basis for future study within the many techniques in current practice.

This is in itself a significant development, though in the event it was only partially successful because, as was reported by Dr Elizabeth Ferris, MB, BS (London), who attended the Congress on behalf of the Psionic Medical Society, most of those present interpreted the aim of the proceedings as a discussion of *alternative* techniques; and as the provisional programme mentioned no less than 135 different therapies, some recognized by orthodoxy, others of a less conventional character, many of the speakers were principally concerned with the advancement of their own particular systems.

As Carl Upton pointed out at the Annual Conference of the Psionic Medical Society in October 1973 (to which Dr Ferris presented her report) any such approach can only lead to greater fragmentation, and hence increasing departure from the truth. Both the established practices of orthodox medicine and the proliferation of so-called fringe techniques are all only partial interpretations of an overriding but unmanifest intelligence of a superior order—the Intelligence which, as mentioned earlier, directs the whole behaviour of the phenomenal world.

We can assume that this was in the minds of the conveners of the Congress, for the very term 'l'Altra Medicina' implies the recognition of a superior level. No real understanding can develop from an assessment of the relative merits of different techniques. Each may have its place, but only as a part of a whole which by its very nature is greater than the sum of its parts; and it is communication with this superior, but incommensurable, whole which provides the key to real knowledge.

Now we have seen that communication with this unmanifest whole is the fundamental basis of psionic medicine. The physical body, and its psychological concomitants, are regarded merely as partial manifestations of the superior pattern which constitutes the whole man; and anyone who has met George Laurence or his colleagues cannot fail to be impressed by their intuitive faith in this reality, and still more by their eminently practical ability to communicate with it.

There are inevitably those who challenge the validity of any phenomena which cannot be explained in terms of logical reasoning. Any effects which fall outside this ambit are either ascribed to imagination, or are assumed to be inexplicable purely because of insufficient knowledge. In their arrogant conceit they are unable to admit the existence of a superior level of intelligence.

There is overwhelming evidence of the existence of phenomena beyond the limits of normal perception. Dowsing is now scientifically accepted, while Dr Lyall Watson discusses a wide range of authenticated paranormal phenomena in his book *Supernature*, all of which confirm that the physical body only provides a very limited interpretation of reality. If one is prepared to throw off the shackles of habitual associations it becomes possible to recognize the practical existence of higher levels of intelligence, which are responsible not only for the ordinary course of events, but also for many phenomena which are customarily regarded as supernatural.

Actually, these effects are only supernatural in terms of the limited intelligence of the senses. To the superior, but dormant, intelligence of the deeper levels of the mind they are entirely natural, and can be utilized. I believe that the practical acknowledgment of these superior influences is an increasingly urgent necessity in the troubled conditions of modern existence, as I have discussed in my book, *The Diary of a Modern Alchemist*. It is all too easy to dismiss the unmanifest realm as abstract speculation, having no relevance to the earnest affairs of life, but this is a lamentably complacent self-deception.

The concept of a hierarchy of levels in the universe provides a glimmer of real understanding. We have discussed the idea of the etheric world as a force-field in which the interplay of influences creates the events and situations in the phenomenal world. This is a disintegrating process, in the sense that by its very multiplicity it is farther removed from the essential unity of the structure; and the modern preoccupation with detail can only result in further departure from unity.

This process would ultimately lead to exhaustion—the dying universe of nineteenth-century science; but it is now realized that the structure is continually revitalized by a return flow of energy towards the source, which is accomplished by process of transformation at every level. Operations within the purely physical realm have a necessary and appropriate importance, but they are entirely circumscribed by physical laws and hence do not produce any change of quality. But there are integrative forces in the universe which can produce transformations of energy from coarser to finer quality. This is real progress, but it can only be achieved by contact with influences of a higher order. These are not subject to physical limitations and can therefore transform the character of the phenomenal manifestations.

By acknowledgment of, and submission to, these superior levels of intelligence, the essential harmony of the human organism can be restored, in part or in whole; but this implies, *ipso facto*, a change of quality, which evidently cannot be achieved to any real extent by manipulation at the physical level only. It is nevertheless possible to communicate with the superior order of intelligence by the exercise of the paranormal senses, as has been shown in the preceding chapters, and it is this communication which forms the basis of homoeopathy and, more precisely, psionic medicine.

Carl Upton has sent me some observations on the relationship between the different approaches. Allopathic medicine, he says, is concerned with the assessment of organic structural and functional derangements, as well as biochemical and psychological imbalances; from which is calculated the physical, biochemical and psychological procedures estimated to correct specific disturbances as and when they occur.

These procedures, however, are often complex, so that their proper co-ordination may be difficult, if not impossible. Moreover, a given procedure, though effective in its original intent, may create undesirable effects in another direction—the so-called 'side effects'—which can be more dangerous, or more tiresome to deal with, than the original complaint.

Neither the diagnosis nor the treatment takes direct account of the vital dynamis, which is the ultimate arbiter of the outcome; and this comprises not only the *Vis Medicatrix Naturae* but the influences of hereditary, racial, family, educational and social factors far beyond the possibility of orthodox allopathic investigation. Account must also be taken of the influence of the environment, including the effects of noise, and the various electromagnetic radiations to which society is subjected. Furthermore, as was well understood by physicians in earlier societies prior to the preoccupation with purely physical science, planetary influences play a vital role in the constitutional make-up of the individual and should not be excluded as a source of psychosomatic imbalance.

The homoeopathic approach to medical problems is more fundamental. It does, of course, take into account both physical symptoms and other circumstantial evidence, but it uses them in a different way. It does not attempt to influence each symptom complex directly, except in emergency where symptomatic interference may be justified temporarily. The homoeopathic physician is interested in the subjective responses of the patient and from this evidence the appropriate homoeopathic medicine is selected, either on the basis of established 'provings' or collected case records; and this of necessity involves the exercise of the intuitive faculty.

It is commonplace in modern medical science to make use of statistical investigation. The outcome is usually a series of 'norms' against which any deviation is assessed; and remedies are prescribed to correct such deviations regardless of the fact that such norms are a pure fiction. Each person has his or her own internal balance or centre of gravity and it is against this that any imbalance must be assessed. So medication should be directed towards this internal imbalance, which is always individual.

Psionic medical philosophy and practice identifies these imbalances by direct perception, making use of the dowsing faculty, thereby disclosing the specific causes of dynamic disturbances of the constitution, and the way in which they may best be removed. This leads to the re-establishment of the individual vital harmony, which is usually effective in removing symptoms provided that irreversible tissue changes have not occurred and overriding inimical influences do not persist in the conditions under which the patient lives.

Psionic medicine is thus essentially an integrating technique; but for this to be exercised it is first necessary to have a sound knowledge of the constituents to be integrated, involving the understanding and experience of established medical principles. This has then to be augmented by personal instruction in the specific techniques of psionic medical practice.

Competence in the use of the pendulum is essential and the British Society of Dowsers has undertaken to train interested doctors and dental surgeons prior to their introduction to the medical applications. Each candidate is then required to attend the Institute of Psionic Medicine in person over a period of time, usually at intervals. The training involves familiarization with charts, samples and witnesses, and with the homoeopathic *Materia Medica*, and then proceeds to the treatment of actual cases.

The courses are arranged individually to minimize the interruption of the practitioner's normal activities, but in view of the demands on the facilities they can only be provided for those who seriously intend to pursue the techniques. I shall be happy to put prospective applicants in touch with the appropriate authorities if they will write to me care of the publishers.

Appendix 1

Simple Exercises with a Pendulum preparatory to Medical Dowsing

Dowsing or divining with a pendulum is an ancient art, but its systematic application as an aid to scientific research or to medical diagnosis and remedy selection is comparatively new.

There is no special power in the pendulum as such. It is simply a convenient instrumental aid, of which the value depends entirely upon the sensitivity of the dowsing faculty of the operator. If this were not so, then a pendulum would react irrespective of the physical contact with the dowser.

A pendulum is, in fact, a simple means of magnifying and rendering visible certain impulses of a biodynamic character, that are activated in the dowser by his paranormal senses.

The pendulum itself, as the name suggests, consists of a weight or bob suspended by thread or fine chain. It can take any form, provided it can be held comfortably by the operator and swing freely above the particular 'field' to be examined.

A length of about 10cm (4in.) is convenient while the bob may be of any material such as glass or plastic. Metal may be used, though it is preferable to use some inert material. The weight is a matter of personal preference. A light bob will provide a rapid response but may be influenced by air currents or unsteadiness of the hand, while a heavy bob may be sluggish in its response. A weight of about 10g ($\frac{1}{3}$oz) is convenient.

It is convenient to attach a short length of chain to the base of the bob since this will provide a clear indication of the path when using a rule or chart. A typical construction is illustrated in figure 3.

Let us now consider the kinds of reaction obtained from the pendulum. There are three basic movements, namely:

1 A simple to-and-fro oscillation usually, but not necessarily, towards and away from the operator;

2 A rotary motion in a clockwise direction;
3 A similar rotary movement anticlockwise.

It is these movements, or combinations thereof, which provide the answers to the questions which are being posed; but there is no hard-and-fast rule. Everyone has to find, by individual experiment, how to interpret the movements. A particular reaction which may indicate to one dowser a certain situation may, to

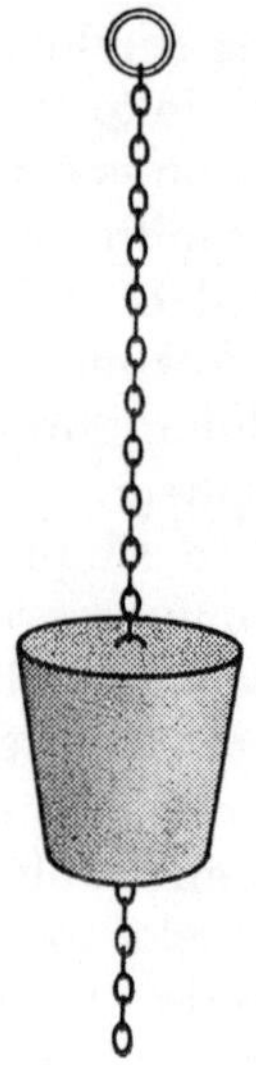

Figure 3
The Dowser's Pendulum

another, suggest the opposite, so that one has to establish by trial one's individual pattern, which with practice will be found to be consistent.

The first requirement is thus to develop the facility for oneself, for which purpose we may commence with a few sample experiments. Sit comfortably at a table on which there is a sheet of white paper, such as a paper tissue. Place on this a pencil, or pen, and hold the pendulum lightly between the thumb and the first (or second) finger over the middle of the object. The hand and arm should be quite relaxed, and it is helpful at the beginning to rest the elbow on the table to keep the hand steady. One should, in fact, be relaxed in body and mind, the mental relaxation being initially the more difficult. One must not expect any particular reaction; but at the same time one must be ready for a response, for if one believes nothing will happen, this very attitude will inhibit any reaction.

After a short time the pendulum will start to oscillate along the length of the pencil. Allow the oscillation to build up to a reasonable swing and then gently move the hand towards the tip of the pencil when the motion will slowly change to a rotation. If the hand is now moved slowly back to the other end of the pencil the pendulum will revert to the oscillating mode until it reaches the end, when it will again rotate, this time in the opposite direction.

At first the pendulum may take a little time to respond. Begin with a length of about 10cm (4in.), but if it is unduly reluctant to start, try altering the length slightly either way. By experiment one soon finds the length best suited to one's personal requirements and with practice it will be found to start swinging almost immediately. However, if there is still no response, wait and try later; one is probably not sufficiently relaxed. In any case, make the attempt alone, for until one has developed the ability, the presence of others is distracting.

One need not be concerned with the reason for this behaviour, for the object of the exercise is merely the acquisition of the basic expertise. In simple terms, any physical object is a local condensation of the etheric force-field, which can be regarded as flowing through the object. With this the pendulum tends to align itself, but at the extremities the field is no longer confined and begins to spread out in all directions, so that the pendulum goes into a gyratory motion. Some exponents of the art pursue this field distribution in detail, but for the present purposes this is neither necessary nor desirable. The pendulum is, in fact, simply answering the mental question 'Is there an object here?'

Even when a response is obtained, do not continue the experiment for more than a brief period, because this creates a tendency to *will* the behaviour of the pendulum, which is very easily done, and can produce spurious indications. It is the initial unconscious reactions which are genuine, and the experiment should be only of brief duration, but repeated at frequent intervals until the reactions occur with increasingly short delay as the facility develops.

A further reason for not prolonging the test is that there is an inherent tendency for the rhythm to change. For example, if the pendulum is gyrating over a sample it will after a certain time change to an oscillation, and after a similar period will revert to gyration in the opposite direction. The number of swings in each mode depends on the substance under examination, and this is utilized by some dowsers to obtain specific information. For the present purpose this is not required and may be ignored, but it is clear that it could confuse the beginner if the test is continued too long.

Another pitfall of which the beginner must be wary is repetition. Finding himself in some doubt about a reading he may be inclined to repeat the procedure, possibly several times. This is to be avoided since it tends to induce a state of mind confusing to the dowsing faculty. The first readings are the most reliable if the mind is clear and the question precise. If there is an overall inconsistency or lack of clarity, all readings should be suspect and it is better to defer further work until mental or other conditions are more favourable.

One can now begin to use the pendulum to answer simple questions. Hold the pendulum over a copper coin of any convenient denomination (or currency) and allow it to build up a gyration. With the free hand touch a second (similar) coin as a 'witness' and observe what happens. Then repeat the experiment with a different witness—e.g. a piece of steel, such as a penknife, or a sample of (genuine) silver, and again observe the reaction.

After a little practice it will be found that in the first case the pendulum will cease to gyrate and will begin to swing to and fro towards the witness, but in the second case it will not alter its mode. This is actually a response to an unconscious inquiry 'Are these two objects of similar material?'—which, of course, one knows to be the case with the two identical coins. With a witness of different material there is no affinity and the pendulum will not change its mode, indicating the answer 'No'.

However, if the experiment is now repeated using a modern so-called silver coin as a witness—e.g. a 5p piece or a dime—the pendulum will again swing towards the witness, suggesting that the coins are of identical material, which they clearly are not. This is a significant example of loose questioning, for in fact both coins contain a predominance of copper and to this extent are of similar constitution; but if one asks mentally, 'Are these coins of *identical* composition?' the pendulum will not deviate, giving a clear answer 'No'.

Given the appropriate knowledge one can discover the actual composition by using as witnesses samples of different (pure) metals, as was discussed in chapter 8, but this need not be elaborated here. The value of this simple experiment lies in its illustration of the need to know precisely what questions to ask; and it is evident that this is absolutely essential in any more sophisticated analysis, particularly of a medical nature.

Water divining is an important and well-known aspect of dowsing and it provides a useful source of experience for the aspirant to medical dowsing. Perhaps the simplest test is to hold the pendulum over a glass of water and after starting an oscillation to watch its subsequent behaviour. As a variant of this exercise the pendulum can first be held a little to one side of the glass and then moved over the glass to the opposite side, noting any change of swing during the process.

Once a consistent reaction has been obtained to the presence of water, further tests can be made over a known water pipe or stream to develop further familiarity with the behaviour of the pendulum. It is then only a short step to water divining proper in its elementary application, namely the location of a hidden underground well or stream, or other location where water is situated.

It will sometimes be noticed that the pendulum gives no response on commencing to dowse. This may occur for a number of reasons but one of the commonest is connected with the distance the pendulum is held away from the object of study. When beginning to dowse, move the pendulum slowly up or down, increasing or decreasing the distance from the object until a response is achieved.

This is a valuable exercise because under different conditions of speed of flow, depth or chemical or bacterial content the pendulum will reflect differences in intensity and speed of swing which can eventually become valuable indicators in medical work.

We now come to a whole series of possibilities for the beginner who has gained some familiarity with the pendulum and its behaviour. We can begin to observe how the pendulum reacts to living tissue.

Hold the pendulum over the back of the lightly clenched fist and observe the swing. Now do the same over the hand of someone of the opposite sex.

Having absorbed the lesson of this simple exercise, smack the back of the hand smartly and watch the reaction of the pendulum again. Repeat the check over the course of half an hour or so and observe any changes in pendulum behaviour that may occur.

Then one may extend the inquiry by watching the reaction of the pendulum to various parts of the body. It will be found probably that not only are there variations in swing in different parts but also between healthy and unhealthy tissue and organs. But of course considerable experience is necessary to be able to interpret such data.

It is very useful to be able to check the vitality of objects that occur in nature. By holding the pendulum above the object under test one can note the type and character of swing and can deduce information of great value. But here it is necessary to frame specific questions with precision.

It is possible to make qualitative evaluations of all manner of material. In the simple testing of a packet of garden seed before planting, or of some fruit or vegetable or other food before eating, one has a most fascinating and useful yardstick to vitality. In these days of devitalized foods this test can become a significant health aid.

Whether a particular item of food is good for one personally or not can also be put to the test. One method, with the question in mind, is to swing the pendulum for a few moments over the back of the hand to get the characteristic reaction and then slowly to move the hand over the food. Any change in swing will indicate whether the food in question is either indifferent or definitely harmful, according to one's personal pendulum convention. Another method is merely to point the index finger of the free hand towards the article to be tested and observe the swing, having of course posed the necessary question.

Poisonous substances may be checked in this way too but it is not advisable to rely upon such a test unless one has considerable experience as a medical dowser.

So far we have been concerned with exercises intended to familiarize the beginner with typical pendulum responses or with straightforward 'yes or no' questions. But in medical dowsing, and particularly in the techniques of psionic medicine, quantitative indications are required. Comparative diagnosis, degree and location of involvement of disease processes and their cause now take place in the dowser's experience.

The pendulum will be called upon to work with two or more witnesses. Devices for recording measurements of degree of pendulum deviation from a point of balance or norm must be introduced. The most usual of these are charts indicating angular deviation and rules for linear measurements.

Two such aids may be considered. The first is the circle and triangle chart used in the Laurence technique of psionic medicine. This chart consists of a circle within a triangle, as illustrated in Figure 4. The radius of the circle is 5cm (2in.), the long side of the triangle being 30cm (12in.), while from the centre of the circle a series of radial lines is drawn at ten degree intervals.

Having constructed such a figure on white paper or card, various exercises can be tried. First place a penny in the right-hand angle of the triangle and in the left a piece of copper wire. Swing the pendulum over the centre of the circle in a to-and-fro motion along the vertical line running through the apex of the triangle and then allow it to take its own course. Observe the degree of any deviation to right or left. Then reverse the positions of coin and copper wire, coin on the left and wire on the right. Once again observe the deviation.

This exercise can be repeated with a variety of objects or with chemicals or foods. It may also be tried with homoeopathic remedies, using different potencies of the same remedy in the right and left angles of the triangle. As a variation, a little saliva on a slip of white blotting paper may be placed on the right-hand angle and tested against various witnesses on the left for possible pendulum deviation. The effect of placing a third object or substance near the apex of the triangle can also be tried.

It is emphasized that these exercises are intended only as a convenient way of getting used to the pendulum in conjunction with a chart. The principle, however, is fundamental to the diagnostic techniques used in psionic medicine.

As a variant to the chart, a ruler may be used to indicate

deviations of various kinds. Take a strip of wood 100cm long and mark it out at 1cm intervals, numbered 50-0-50. The two 50 marks then take the place of the left and right angles of the triangle in the chart just described.

Exercises may then be tried by placing witnesses on these

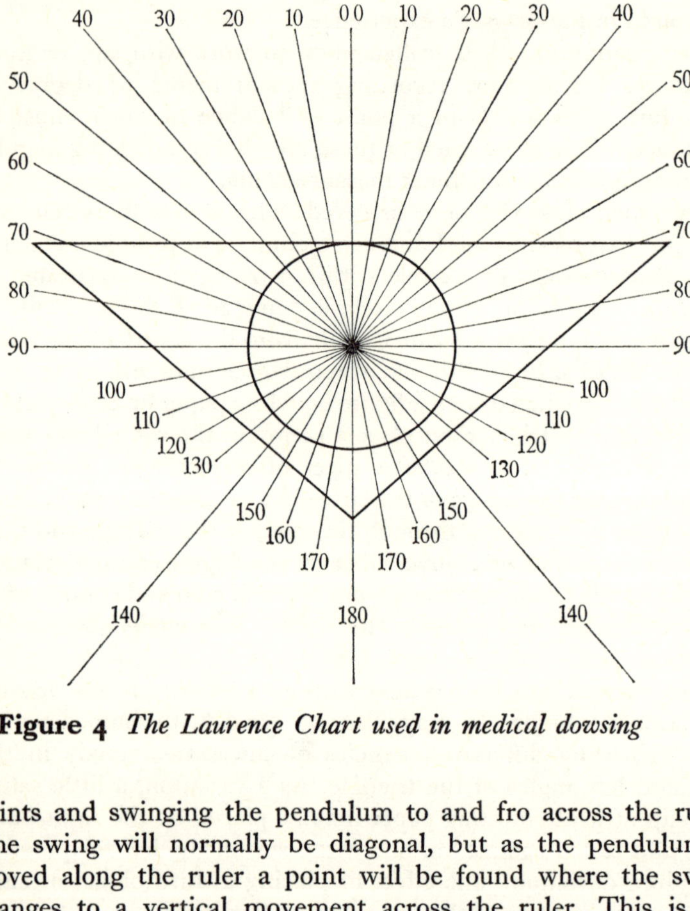

Figure 4 *The Laurence Chart used in medical dowsing*

points and swinging the pendulum to and fro across the ruler. The swing will normally be diagonal, but as the pendulum is moved along the ruler a point will be found where the swing changes to a vertical movement across the ruler. This is the balance point from which the desired information may be deduced.

These various exercises will serve to introduce the aspirant to the art of dowsing in order to develop a certain facility with the pendulum. The student should record his reactions with a view to establishing a coherent pattern of response. He can then begin to devise for himself various extensions and modifications to increase his experience, and try to co-ordinate his conclusions.

At this stage it becomes possible to develop the faculty more precisely, but for this, particularly in any attempts at medical dowsing, it is necessary to seek expert instruction.

Appendix 2

Commentary by George Laurence on McDonagh's Unitary Concept of Disease

The essence of McDonagh's theory is that there is only one disease, and that it arises from the protein in the blood being so affected that it can no longer properly fulfil its original function of attracting food, storing it in itself, and then radiating it to the tissues and organs in a balanced way.

All so-called diseases are merely manifestations of imbalance or aberration of the protein, and no disease can be cured unless that balance is restored. McDonagh points out that you may palliate or alleviate manifestations of disease, you can suppress and drive them from one place to another (e.g. the alternation of skin disease and asthma as the result of treatment directed solely to one or the other manifestation), and you can keep them hidden for long periods, but you cannot cure them unless you can find the basic cause or common denominator. However perfect a chemotherapeutic preparation may be, it can never be relied upon to remove all the lesions and effect the disappearance of all such manifestations, as its sole action is to repair the local secondary damage suffered by the protein; and as it has no effect whatsoever upon the primary cause or causes of the damage, that repair may be of a very temporary nature. This is a point of the importance of which orthodox medicine seems to be generally sublimely oblivious —or indifferent!

The real question before us is: why is there a primary protein imbalance? Infection by micro-organisms may come to mind and steps be taken to destroy them biochemically; but in killing them, have you found the reason why the individual became in the first place so vulnerable to attack? Why is health so undermined as to permit the invasion? Or again, as many of us are beginning to wonder, what is amiss with our mental or spiritual outlook, or with our food and environment, that the resistance of our tissues is so low?

To get nearer the answer to our question it seems necessary to consider the nature of health; and to arrive at this we must realize that an important part of its origin lies in the soil. Micro-organisms, by their action on other micro-organisms and the mineral and plant life, liberate vital energies which constitute the principal ingredient of the nourishment extracted by plants from the soil. Hence a deficiency of life in the soil means inferior quality of food for plants and consequent inferiority of food for animals, and so for men, whether taken in animal or vegetable form.

To quote McDonagh, 'The soil beneath our feet is not simply a dead, inert mass, but is composed of countless millions of living organisms, each with its own tiny life cycle and particular work to perform. Healthy vital bodies require vital foods grown upon living soil. Yet what do we find? Sick bodies and minds and uncontrolled emotions, fed upon devitalised foods which have been raised upon sick, tired and worn-out soil.'

Thus an important factor of health is the state of the soil and there is a link here with protein aberrations in the body. It is encouraging to note, therefore, that the question of soil is at last getting some consideration particularly in regard to the deficiencies that we have to contend with in treatment of both acute and chronic disease.

Climate and proper food are the fundamental requirements for the soil and its micro-organisms, and when conditions exist such as an unsuitable climate, exhaustion of the soil or ill-treatment by chemical fertilizers or insecticides and weedkillers, the micro-organisms are unable to do their work properly and thus our food suffers. We have no control over climate and, as individuals, very little over the quality of the food that is offered to us, but we can be much more careful in our choice of food. If the public demand for wholemeal flour, brown sugar and cereals, fruit and vegetables grown on compost-cultivated soil, clean milk, unadulterated and genuine food, became sufficiently clamant, there would be an enormous decrease in chronic disease and an improvement in the health of the nation.

In addition to the intestinal toxaemia caused by contaminated and unsuitable food, there are, of course, a large number of other causes of chronic disease—occupational, psychological and environmental—to which must be added the debilitating effects of the miasms discussed in chapter 5. All of these influences create disturbance of the balance of the protein so that in this sense there is, as McDonagh affirms, only one disease.

McDonagh maintains that under the influence of 'climate', which I understand to mean cosmic energy, all protein alternately expands and contracts, and if the extent and rhythm of this pulsation is upset—rendered aberrant, to use his own term—you have a state of imbalance and the condition necessary to produce disease.

He divides protein into three portions corresponding to and exercising the three main developmental divisions of the body. These he calls the Epiblast, the Mesoblast and the Hypoblast, which should operate in harmony.

Very briefly, McDonagh derives from the mesoblast:

Musculo-skeletal system	Genito-urinary system
Cardio-vascular system	Adrenal cortex

From the hypoblast:

Blood	Thyroid
Respiratory system	Portal system

From the epiblast:

Adrenal medulla	Sympathetic nervous system
Anterior pituitary	Parasympathetic
Posterior pituitary	nervous system

The clinical symptoms may differ according to which portions of the protein are mostly thrown out of balance, but as you cannot confine a toxin to one portion of the body, you generally have to deal with the whole picture in the first place.

From a sample of the patient such as a spot of blood, saliva or hair, or even a photograph or signature, a considerable amount of information about the state of protein can be obtained by the use of a pendulum in experienced hands—quite unbelievable, of course, to the uninitiated and orthodox fraternity; this I can well understand, for when I first heard of radiesthesia, I was similarly sceptical. But the technique is now scientifically established, and I find it sad that so many people are suffering unnecessarily for want of informed treatment beyond the scope of the more or less casual administration of synthetic chemicals, so many of which are poisonous because they cause further imbalance of the protein;

and this despite the fact that they can produce only temporary alleviation or suppression of symptoms.

By the use of the pendulum it is possible to find out, with the aid of witnesses, whether a toxin is present, what it is and its extent, and what particular part of the body is mostly being affected. As a poison cannot be confined to one place (think of a snake bite, or even a sting), it is neither sensible nor even intelligent to treat any specific effect before removing the cause. Once you have dealt with the primary cause, you can treat such symptoms as are still left with the ordinary homoeopathic remedies and so redress any secondary aberration of the protein in the individual organs.

The principle of first finding the basic cause of any malady applies with special force to chronic disease. I could give many examples of this, but an outstanding one is afforded by many cases of alternating asthma and eczema which I have been seeing for myself during some sixty years of practice. Both chest specialists and dermatologists can give temporary relief to one or other manifestation, often causing an exacerbation of the untreated symptom, but neither knowing what is really the matter with the patient nor ascertaining the basic cause.

It seems to me quite wrong to accept a name or a label as a true diagnosis. Surely that term should include the cause; otherwise it can only claim to be a provisional diagnosis. Another example is migraine, the treatment of which seems to be much on the same lines as when I was a student, whereas the underlying cause can be different in different people. Until that cause is removed, you can again only expect temporary relief by drugs—with the very definite risk of serious side effects.

So many of these chronic diseases are due to inherited miasms or acquired toxins which remain in the body, and these can only be detected by supersensory methods. The outlook for the effective handling of such cases appears to be very grim, unless the value of psionic techniques for diagnosis and treatment becomes more widely recognized.

It is little short of amazing how, with a little practice, the pendulum will pick out the appropriate remedy, and moreover tell you quite definitely which potency is likely to be the most effective. This is of especial value, as in orthodox homoeopathic teaching the question of potencies is always a stumbling block and depends very much on the personal preference or experience of the practitioner. Furthermore, the pendulum can give you a very good idea of the exact dosage and the length of time for which the remedy should be prescribed.

To recapitulate, the basic structure of the body consists of protein, for which the fats and carbohydrates act mostly as fuel. Any condition which disturbs the harmonious balance of the protein causes ill-health, of which the manifestations and symptoms depend upon what region or regions of the protein are suffering the imbalance.

In my own practice the great proportion of cases before I see them have been subjected to the most exhaustive—and often exhausting—investigations, clinical, laboratory, Barium meals, X-rays, etc., with negative results, and patients have come to see me as a last hope. It is quite wonderful how frequently psionic techniques will provide not only a true diagnosis but also an effective treatment, especially in the case of the so-called incurable diseases, of which the basic cause has so seldom been found.

I owe a debt of gratitude to McDonagh for the light he has thrown on the problem of medicine and very much regret that so few orthodox doctors will even try to understand what he means by his unitary theory, much less apply it to the elucidation of the problem of disease and use it for the alleviation of human suffering.

Appendix 3

Clinical Cases

In this appendix will be found a number of examples of conditions in which the orthodox approach has achieved little or no success, but which have responded, in some cases dramatically, to the treatment by psionic medical techniques of the underlying causes.

For convenience, they are grouped where possible under specific headings. Some cases in the various categories have been discussed in chapter 13.

1 Migraine

Case 5 Mr S. C. W. S., aged 44

The patient reported that he had had frequent attacks of migraine over 25 years, latterly several times a week. He also complained of continual tiredness. The first signs of an attack were flashing lights on one side, followed by pain over one eye. This was followed by pain down the side of the head, a feeling of sickness and then vomiting on most occasions. Whilst an attack was in progress there was a dislike of bright light. The duration of the attack was usually about five hours.

A psionic diagnosis revealed the double tubercular miasm and a meningeal imbalance. There was also a measles toxin. Treatment was started with a view to eliminating inherited and acquired toxic factors and an immediate reduction in frequency and intensity of attack occurred. Five months later the patient wrote to say, 'I have now finished my last course of tablets. Since my last report to you I am pleased to tell you that I have had no attacks of migraine at all.'

Case 6 Mrs R. J., housewife, aged 41

This patient complained of severe headache with nausea, both at her periods and midway between, from the age of 20. She was also subject to states of great depression and extreme agitation.

As a child she had hay fever for which she had injections, also measles at 18, and German measles at 34. There was a poor family history. She had all the usual allopathic treatments, but was steadily getting worse. The psionic analysis of her blood sample gave readings on TB/TK miasms and also an acquired measles toxin.

The indicated treatment was started but near the end had to be discontinued as she suddenly felt very ill, and was diagnosed by the family doctor as having influenza. A psionic diagnosis showed no sign of this, but a very toxic liver, which was corrected by a dose of podophyllin 1M.

When she was well again a further psionic check-up was made and this showed that the first treatment had been effective in spite of the interruption. Both miasms and the toxin had been eliminated. Treatment was then started to deal with the after-effects, principally an adrenal cortex deficiency and an imbalance on the autonomic nervous system. She reported in due course that she felt fine, no headaches, and more energy and vitality, and much less depressed.

Case 7 Mrs D. J., housewife and mother, aged 38

This patient had suffered from migraines since she was 15, and had been taking Migril and Conovid E for the last four years, which made her feel sick and bad tempered. She also found that of late she was getting mental and emotional disturbances and life was becoming a misery.

A psionic analysis showed that she had both TB/TK miasms and an acquired measles toxin, and that the drugs had reduced her general vitality very seriously. These were therefore stopped and psionic treatment substituted. After a short period of homoeopathic aggravation she began to settle down, and by the time she finished the first course of treatment she was feeling much better in every way.

A check-up showed a remarkable improvement and she was only given stabilizing treatment. She continued to improve and even lost the headache she had always had during menstruation. Indeed she felt so much better that she had left off treatment.

However she had a relapse and tension headaches returned, so treatment was recommenced, as she was found psionically to have various vitamin and mineral deficiencies. This was corrected, and there has been no recurrence now for over two years.

Case 8 Mrs X., housewife and mother, aged 45

This patient had severe migraines since she started to menstruate at 13, together with various other allergies, for which she had tried every form of treatment with no lasting relief.

She proved to be a very difficult case to treat, as the basic cause was found to be three hereditary miasms (including the double tubercular miasms) which were very difficult to dislodge; in fact it was not until she had had five courses of basic treatment that the miasms were finally eliminated.

There were homoeopathic aggravations but on the whole the symptoms slowly became less severe, until four months after commencing treatment she could report she hoped she had turned the corner.

Treatment was continued off and on for another six months, by which time she was very much better in every way. She has had treatment for other minor ailments which have cropped up as a result of foreign travel, but the original migraines and allergic symptoms are now a thing of the past.

Case 9 Mr J. W., aged 20

This case is typical of many migraine sufferers, both symptomatically and causatively. The patient complained of frequent and severe attacks of headache and photophobia, usually at weekly intervals. The attack lasted for one or two days and was accompanied by the characteristic nausea. There were no other outstanding symptoms apart from a high incidence of dental caries.

Psionic analysis revealed both tubercular miasms and activity of sycotic co., a non-lactose fermenting bowel organism usually associated with the catarrhal state.

Treatment was initiated to remove the miasms and the toxin, and the response was rapid, the symptoms subsiding within a few weeks. A little later the patient contracted influenza, which was given appropriate homoeopathic treatment and which led to a short period in the negative phase, with characteristic feeling of tiredness and depression. Some three months after the first treatment for the removal of the miasms some bronchial symptoms appeared, and these were found to be associated with staphylococcus aureus infection. When this was cleared the patient required no further treatment and has remained well and symptom-free since.

2 Brucellosis

A particularly intractable problem today is that of brucellosis which, either in the form of brucella abortus or brucella melitensis, is causing increasing concern in the medical and veterinary world. Its effect in cattle is well known, where it seems to be replacing the now largely eliminated bovine TB.

Its incidence in humans, usually known as undulant or Malta fever, is very difficult to treat by orthodox methods. The symptoms can be alleviated, but tend to recur, so that a condition of poor health may continue for years with little hope of definite cure. The following cases illustrate how psionic treatment can provide rapid and permanent release.

Case 10 Mrs M. M., farmer's wife, aged 46

In the spring of 1965 the family bought a house cow giving a plentiful supply of milk and cream. By July Mrs M. M. had developed headaches, marked tiredness, sweating at night, with a slight evening temperature—subnormal in the morning. In August an orthodox blood test gave a diagnosis of brucellosis. The infected milk was eliminated and she was given a course of antibiotics, but warned that there might be a recurrence. This proved to be the case as from then onwards she was up and down but always below par, tired and lacking in energy.

By October 1968 her condition had definitely deteriorated with continual tiredness, night sweats, headaches and lassitude. In January 1969 she came under psionic treatment. Analysis of a blood spot gave a high reading on brucella melitensis, and all systems of the body were affected, particularly the musculo-skeletal, the portal, and the central and autonomic nervous systems, the adrenal cortex, the thyroid and the pineal, with a low general vitality reading.

She was given the psionically-indicated homoeopathic treatment lasting for three weeks, which resulted in the total elimination of the brucella infection and an almost complete restoration of normality to the body as a whole, only necessitating a simple holding homoeopathic prescription for eighteen days. No further treatment was required, and, up to date, report is that the patient has not felt so well and full of energy for years, with no sign of recurrence of symptoms of any sort.

Case 11 Miss Y., aged 46

In April 1961 this patient complained of spots on the face and ulcers on the tongue, and, in July, of epigastric discomfort and more spots on the face. In March 1962 she had great discomfort in the eyelids and patches on the forehead and near the mouth. She now became more and more allergic, particularly to plants which, as she was a great gardener, she found most distressing. During April she complained of intermittent urticaria, nettlerash, etc., and in May she developed an angio-neurotic oedema. For all this she was given ordinary symptomatic treatment.

At the beginning of September she had four severe attacks of acute urticaria in the space of ten days, and sought the help of a psionic medical practitioner. A blood-spot analysis gave a marked brucellosis reaction and a sample of the farm milk she was drinking also gave a reaction. An interesting point was that her mother and sister were also drinking the same milk with no ill effects.

The farmer from whom she obtained the milk scoffed at the diagnosis in regard to his milk and refused to accept its validity. But it was found that the milk came from two sources, ordinary cows and Jersey cows, which latter gave no reaction. When the patient only drank the Jersey milk she began to recover and then with the appropriate psionic treatment for brucellosis all her allergic symptoms cleared up and she made a complete recovery and remained healthy.

Case 12 Mr T. B., stockman, aged 43

This patient was in charge of a herd of goats, certified to be free from TB and brucellosis, and he had not been in contact with cows. However, he became ill and was diagnosed as a case of brucellosis.

He was sent into hospital where he was treated with streptomycin by daily injection. On this treatment he went deaf, so the medicine was changed to deal with the side effect, but this new treatment upset his stomach, so again it had to be altered; and still without change in the brucella condition. He was off work for about eleven weeks, and was told it would probably be a year before he was really better.

At this point he came under psionic medical care and was given a course of treatment at the end of which a hospital blood test was said to show 'marked improvement'. A further test after a second course of psionic treatment was pronounced to be 'very satisfactory', and there was no further recurrence of the symptoms.

3 Asthma and Allied Conditions

This is a complaint particularly prevalent in children, often accompanied by eczema. Its causes are often deep-seated requiring prolonged homoeopathic medication but psionic treatment is ultimately successful.

Case 13 M. H., male, aged 9½

This was a young boy who had been troubled with asthma and recurring eczema since the age of 6 months. It was not until he was 9½ that his parents sought the advice of a psionic practitioner, who discovered two underlying miasms—TK and polio. After two and a half months the polio miasm was eliminated, and the TK miasm greatly reduced, but a TB miasm was then uncovered, together with one of pertussis.

The indicated treatment was given for a further six months, but although the pertussis miasm disappeared at once, and the readings of the TK and TB were reduced, the miasms remained remarkably resistant; and it was not until March (1967) that they were cleared. But he then developed a staph. aur. infection and, surprisingly, the miasms became active for a further two months before disappearing completely.

During a year at school, during the earlier part of which he was having continuous treatment, his health improved considerably and he had no time off, but on returning home for the summer holidays his wheeziness returned. This was assumed to be due to emotional excitement, but after further homoeopathic treatment it subsided, and on his Christmas holiday there was no recurrence, despite an influenza epidemic at the time.

In February 1968 his father wrote, 'It is very apparent that the treatment given my son has been progressively successful in its results. His health is now excellent and he has not lost any time from school, whilst he is acquitting himself well academically and more than holding his own with the other boys.'

This case brings out an important fact, namely that in these deep-seated chronic conditions, even though the underlying causal factors are eliminated, a residual pattern appears to remain temporarily, and this can be activated by extraneous toxic and emotional factors, as in this case, where emotion could bring on the attacks of wheeziness.

Case 14 N. T., male, aged 7

This child had had asthma practically all his life; he continually missed school and was a great worry to his mother who could do little for his obvious distress.

Psionic diagnosis in September 1966 showed the usual TB/TK miasms together with a measles toxin. After two courses of treatment his mother reported at the end of October that he had had no colds and no return of the asthma, whereas previously a cold always produced a severe attack. He has not looked back, and his mother says that the cure has changed both their lives.

Case 15 F. M. H., female, aged 60

This patient had suffered attacks of asthma since she was about 44 years old, with increasing intensity. A delicate child, with a tendency to chest trouble, she complained of constant breathlessness and recurrent bronchitis. Constipation and increase of girth at diaphragm level were also featured. There was incipient cataract. Operations for the removal of gall bladder and appendix had been performed.

A psionic medical analysis was carried out in November 1968 and this indicated the presence of the double tubercular miasm together with the acquired toxins resulting from streptococcus infection and malaria. A later analysis showed the patient to be sensitive to aluminium used in cooking.

Several courses of homoeopathic medicines were necessary, the final course being in April 1969, when an atypical bacillus coli bowel organism was present. After this was cleared the patient reported a good state of general health and complete freedom from asthma and chest trouble. The improvement has been maintained.

This case illustrates the diversity of symptoms that can occur through the presence of mixed miasms and acquired toxins. It also shows how in some cases the final response of the organism in cure produces changes in the bowel flora; and once this is corrected the case proceeds to a satisfactory conclusion.

Case 16 Mrs I. C., aged 49

This was a case of chronic dermatitis of arms and legs which failed to respond to orthodox medical treatment. Various forms of skin lesions were present, prescribed for both by general medical practitioner and by hospital skin specialist over a period of three years without effect. As the patient was engaged in domestic work using detergents it was thought that this might have a bearing and protective gloves were advised but with no effect. Cortisone ointment was given but on other advice this was discontinued because of side effects. The trouble appeared to be spreading and the patient became desperate.

On the advice of her employer she agreed to psionic medical analysis. This showed that inherited miasms of syphilis and tuberculosis were present as well as the toxins of staphylococcus and aluminium. The indicated homoeopathic medicines were prescribed and there was an immediate improvement. After three courses of medicines all lesions had completely cleared and the skin was perfectly normal. The patient throughout had continued her domestic work. Two years later the skin remains normal.

Case 17 M. S.-R., female, aged 6¾

This child had measles at 20 months and bronchitis when she was two years old, followed shortly afterwards by a further attack, and a month later, pneumonia.

Thereafter she had recurring attacks of bronchial asthma. Every cold always seemed to develop into this, and was only relieved by Wright's Coal Tar Vaporizer, and 'Alupent'. Each attack would last for about a week, and she was frequently rushed to hospital.

When she was nearly seven, in August, further advice was sought. A psionic diagnosis showed that the underlying factors of her illness were TK/TB miasms and the acquired measles toxin. The indicated treatment was given which at first increased the asthma (homoeopathic aggravation), but she quickly recovered. With further treatment the miasms and toxin factors disappeared, and by January, in spite of a bad cold in November, she became free from her asthma and was in good health and has remained so.

Case 18 G. C., male, aged 15

At the age of two he had an attack of acute bronchitis and thereafter suffered from repeated attacks of chest complaints until he was seven. He was finally taken to a specialist as his mother was convinced he was an asthmatic. This was confirmed and Ephedrine etc. prescribed, and for a while the attacks diminished in frequency, but increased in severity and he did not appear to recover so quickly after an attack.

As he got older the doctor's dictum that 'he would grow out of it' did not seem to be happening; rather the reverse, as he was undersized for his age and could not take part in school games or sports due to breathlessness on exertion. Therefore, when he was fifteen, his mother, now very concerned about his condition, sought further advice from a psionic practitioner. Clinical examination showed no signs in the chest and expansion was fair, but he was pale, thin and underdeveloped.

Psionic diagnosis showed there was an asthmatic condition due to the miasms of TK and of whooping cough. So in April he was given the appropriate treatment which eliminated the whooping cough miasms and reduced the TK reading.

The following check-up, however, now revealed an acquired measles toxin. This was dealt with and the TK reading still further reduced, but it took three further courses of treatment to eliminate the TK miasm completely. During this time, however, he was making good progress both generally and with the asthmatic condition, apart from an easily induced wheeziness. But he did not gain in weight.

However, after a further seven months of treatment by November he became completely free of all miasms and toxic factors, and thereafter only required treatment to consolidate his newly acquired health.

By March, a year after starting treatment, his health was excellent. There were no signs of asthma, not even a cold, and he was filling out and beginning to look his age. In due course he went on from his grammar school to university and now plays rugby.

Case 19 W. L., female, $11\frac{1}{2}$ in April 1962

When she was first seen by the psionic practitioner, she was so short of breath she could not come into the consulting room, but had to stay outside by the window.

She had had skin trouble from 3 months old and asthma from the age of one year. The psionic analysis gave a very high reading on the TB/TK miasms and a strong measles 'hangover', so no wonder the child was ill.

With treatment she was soon easier, and by May much better. By July she only had occasional attacks of wheezing, and by August was practically well, but her skin took a great deal longer to clear up, and even now at 15 tends to eliminate any infection via her skin, but fortunately this generally yields fairly soon to treatment.

Case 20 L. B., female, aged 13
Irritability, occasional asthma attacks, intermittent bowel looseness and adenoids were the symptoms complained of in this child. Psionic medical analysis showed the existence of the tubercular miasms. This was in July 1966.

Treatment for the removal of the miasms was undertaken with a rapid response. In October 1967 there was a return of the asthma. A further analysis showed that one of the tubercular miasms had not been completely eliminated and this was obviously the cause of the recurrence. Suitable treatment resulted in a return to normal.

On two occasions since then the patient has caught a cold and this has resulted in some chest difficulty, but each time there has been a favourable response to the homoeopathic medicines prescribed. The history does, however, show that in some cases, despite the removal of miasms, there is a typical symptom pattern that can be triggered off if a minor infection occurs. Possibly this was marked in this child because of the fact that the mother suffered an active tubercular infection at the time she was carrying the child; incidentally, the mother was cured of the tuberculosis by homoeopathic medicines prescribed on psionic medical indications and is now perfectly fit and well. Family difficulties and the emotional stresses aroused also appeared to be a trigger cause of asthmatic attacks in this child.

4 Allergies and Aluminium Sensitivity

Affections of the skin are of frequent occurrence and are often difficult to diagnose. They may be due to allergic conditions but in many instances are the result of toxins acquired from the inimical energies in aluminium utensils, as was discussed in chapter 5. Examples of both forms are given below.

Case 21 Mrs D. M., aged 40

The complaint in this case was recurring patches of dry skin, especially on the face, which sometimes became red and irritable. The onset was usually quite unexpected and rapid. There was also at the same time a persistent breakdown of the skin at the margin of the nostrils on one side with unpleasant ulceration. The eye was also sometimes affected. There were no miasms or toxins associated with infectious illness since these had all been removed previously. A further, rather wider analysis showed that the patient was sensitive to cat hair. Accordingly, during an attack, potentized cat hair was prescribed as the remedy and at the second dose the skin cleared completely.

After several weeks, however, there was a further eruption with similar skin characteristics. On this occasion a further dose of cat hair failed to be effective. A yet more comprehensive analysis showed a sensitivity to primula and indeed it was confirmed that a primula was present in the house. Attention having been drawn to this new possibility careful observation showed that in fact when the primula was touched there was an immediate skin reaction. Homoeopathic primula was prescribed and the plant removed. There have been no further complaints. This illustrates the fact that when the basic constitutional predispositions are eliminated it does not necessarily follow that residual effects are clear. They may persist and require attention for some time.

Case 22 Mrs W. T., aged 40

This patient had suffered from a chronic area of ulceration on her right leg for three years. This did not respond to any form of orthodox medication applied. She had a yellowish complexion and said that she had a history of pyelitis for ten years. She also complained of an eye lesion which was said to be of tropical origin.

Psionic medical diagnosis revealed the presence of the double tubercular inherited miasm, acquired toxins of bacillus coli, and aluminium poisoning. Appropriate treatment was commenced and the patient was advised to discard her aluminium kitchenware, which she had been using extensively. There was a good response to the initial medication which was continued at intervals with further improvement. After four months the patient reported complete recovery with no vestige of the former skin condition.

Case 23 Mrs J. McC., aged 60

This patient was undergoing treatment from her general practitioner and from a specialist at a general hospital. The most serious aspect of her condition appeared to be that she was suffering from repeated 'blackouts' and drug intoxication from the many medicines that had been prescribed. But apart from this she was completely undermined by a severe skin rash which extended over the whole of the face and neck apart from other parts of the body. The rash took the form of a white mass of scales with a red and irritant base. The effect was quite hideous and a source of embarrassment both to the patient and to the family.

Various forms of treatment had failed to bring any improvement. It was pointed out to the patient that since she was already receiving medication of various kinds it was not possible to go into her case and prescribe until such medication had been completed. However, it was agreed to make a preliminary psionic analysis, which immediately indicated that the skin condition was related to aluminium poisoning which could be treated quite simply by giving two tablets with a 24-hour interval between them and would not interfere with any general medication. Three days later the patient phoned to say that a miracle had occurred. All the scales had fallen off and the skin base was resolving fast. In a few more days the face appeared normal and no further trouble has been experienced.

Case 24 Mr I. B. M. C., aged 56

In this case there had been a colon imbalance for twelve years. It was originally associated with a pain in the groin and testicles. He had some symptoms of migraine. His appetite was small. He had a history of diphtheria as a child.

Psionic analysis showed the double tubercular miasm, the acquired toxins of measles and aluminium. Three prescriptions were given between June 1972 and the end of August with good results. The patient, who had been using aluminium extensively, changed all utensils in the kitchen to enamel and stainless steel. He also took precautions as far as possible to avoid aluminium factory preparations in the form of processed foods, and whenever possible avoided likely bearers of the toxins when eating out.

At the beginning of November the patient noted a little digestive upset of a temporary nature. Analysis revealed the recurrence of aluminium toxins. Powders were prescribed and the patient wrote: 'I think we have the answer to the renewed aluminium poisoning. As the fresh vegetables from the garden have come to an end for the season, we have been drawing on our supplies from the freezer, and in using those packets of earlier date we used some that had been put down last year. This means that they were treated before freezing in our old pressure cooker made of aluminium. They were so treated, of course, before I went to you in the first place and learned of my sensitivity to the metal. So now I shall use none of our frozen stuff until we reach the date of our change of kitchen ware.'

5 Miscellaneous conditions

We will conclude with examples of a wide variety of conditions, some straightforward, others less well defined, in which psionic techniques have proved effective.

Case 25 Mrs E. P., aged 44. Schizophrenia

This patient had a record of outbursts of vituperation and violence. In 1966 when she was 41, she started a transport business, which grew so rapidly she became heavily overburdened with problems and in 1968 she had a mental breakdown, becoming withdrawn, intent on psychic matters and spiritualism, with various psychotic manifestations and symptoms which were finally diagnosed as schizophrenia. But by this time she had so lost touch with reality that she had landed herself and her husband in a crippling debt. Her condition deteriorated and by January 1970 she took to her bed with fantasies and delusions of her identity. She was finally taken to a mental hospital but refused treatment and left after two days.

Her husband in desperation asked for homoeopathic treatment on psionic medical indications. The diagnosis of her bloodspot showed both syphilitic and tubercular miasms particularly affecting her brain and central nervous system, but in addition she had an atypical bacillus coli in the bowel (probably the result of previous use of antibiotics), and cellular dehydration.

The treatment indicated and prescribed was in four stages but administration proved very difficult and at times appeared hopeless as the patient chain-smoked, drank tea and coffee as well as wine at the time of taking the remedies, regardless of advice to the contrary, and later refused all treatment at two periods midway between the second and third stages.

In April she became unmanageable and suicidal and was forcibly removed to a mental hospital where she remained for a month and improved under conventional treatment. On returning home she refused all treatment and began to drink heavily once more. She deteriorated rapidly and again took to her bed. But at this point she suddenly agreed to resume the homoeopathic treatment and the third stage was completed, but she continued to drink as she could not sleep.

The fourth stage of treatment however was now commenced on 6 August. After the first powder of this she went to bed, slept soundly, and in succeeding days drank less, continued to sleep well, and on 21 August after the sixth powder she stated she felt she had passed the crisis.

She continued to improve all round and by the end of August went with her small son and her mother to the south coast, and her husband joining them for the weekend found her 'healthy, cheerful and normal'; by September a psionic check-up showed she was at last clear of all miasms and toxic factors.

From this point she gradually moved stage by stage back to ordinary normal life, in spite of the fact that in doing so she would be facing a disastrous financial situation. Her humour and quick intelligence returned. She became increasingly physically active and her husband stated 'that the change is so striking as to make the past year or two seem unreal'.

At the present time (mid-March 1971) she remains perfectly normal and orientated. She has just completed the restoration of a farm house, taking full responsibility for the planning and supervision of structural alterations. She has taken up business affairs again and her old hobbies, particularly painting. She has completely left her illness and all it stood for behind her.

Case 26 Mrs Y. Hodgkin's disease

As a little girl of eight, she was diagnosed, after most careful investigations, as a case of Hodgkin's disease, and her parents were told by the hospital that there was nothing more they could do for her and it was only a matter of time. In view of this hopeless prognosis the parents turned to psionic medicine, and a diagnosis made showed heavy readings on TB/TK hereditary miasms. The indicated treatment was given and the child made a complete recovery.

She is now a healthy wife and mother of a very fit five-year-old daughter.

Case 27 W. N., male, aged 10. Physical and mental retardation
From the age of three this boy suffered from throat and ear trouble, and was about a year behind others of his age in every way. His tonsils and adenoids were removed with no improvement, and finally his parents were told by the ENT specialist that he had an allergic condition and would suffer from such troubles all his life.

When he was seven a psionic analysis showed the cause of his trouble to be TB/TK hereditary miasms and an acquired measles toxin. The indicated homoeopathic treatment was started and continued at intervals for some time. The result has been that the ear and throat trouble was completely cleared, and he has been completely free ever since. His mental and physical slowness which had been such a worry also steadily improved, and he is now holding his own at school with boys of his own age.

Case 28 D. J., female, aged 7. Coeliac disease
This little girl had suffered ill-health from birth and was diagnosed as a case of coeliac disease. Under expert medical treatment it was found that she could not eat anything made with wheat flour, and the specialist advised her parents that she would always require a gluten-free diet and that great care would have to be taken all her life. In July 1970 she came under psionic medical treatment. The diagnosis showed she had the double TB/TK miasm, as well as the acquired measles toxin. She was given the indicated homoeopathic treatment, and by September all her symptoms had completely cleared up, and she was able to eat anything. She has remained completely normal since.

Case 29 F. R., male, aged 47. Liver disorder
This patient had been ailing for over a year with recurrent attacks of jaundice and pain over the liver region. He had been seen by a

specialist who appeared to be somewhat baffled, but thought a liver cancer was a possibility and suggested he went into hospital for further investigation including liver biopsy.

At this point he came under psionic medical attention and on a diagnosis being made this showed the trouble was an infection with a nosode-sycotic co. There was no sign of precancer or cancer readings, which finding was reinforced by a normal reading on the anterior pituitary.

The indicated treatment was first one powder of sycotic co, 10M; but it was not possible to get this until four days after the psionic analysis, and during this period his symptoms became worse and he had to take to his bed. But on the morning of the fifth day he took the high potency powder, with the following result in his own words: 'By late afternoon I had more pain, but was better in myself, especially round the region of the eyes. The marked improvement continued so that now I feel better than at any time since twelve months ago. The pain over the liver disappeared altogether by the sixth day after taking the powder, and except for a few twinges from time to time I have become progressively better.'

A check-up was made at the end of this treatment and showed a normal state of affairs except for a slight anaemia, which was treated. There has been no relapse and the patient's health has remained excellent.

Case 30 N. C., male, aged 68. General debility

This patient had over a period of some four months been running an intermittent temperature, sometimes as high as 102 degrees, with rigors, nausea and vomiting. He was becoming anaemic, with loss of weight, urinary trouble and constipation.

At the hospital he had numerous blood tests and X-rays of abdomen and chest with no positive findings. The diagnosis to start with had been influenza, later more serious possibilities; but no final diagnosis was made and no treatment given except purely symptomatic.

He finally took things into his own hands and went on a fruit and vegetable diet and sought the help of psionic medicine. The psionic diagnosis revealed a double TB/TK miasm plus an acquired measles toxin, but also a precancer reading. Apart from the respiratory system and the thyroid all the systems and organs of the body were considerably affected, particularly the blood, liver and the anterior pituitary and adrenal cortic. The prognosis looked grave.

However, treatment was started. After a week he reported that he already felt better, though he thought this might be due to the fact that the cause was now known and treatment had been started. But after a further fortnight he said he still felt better and more his old self.

A psionic check-up when the treatment was finished showed a marked improvement in the readings. His general vitality had gone up, and all the systems and organs had improved considerably. The miasmic and toxic factors had completely gone but there was still a small precancer reading and a phosphorus deficiency (a usual finding after elimination of miasms and toxins).

Follow-up treatment was given, and he continued to improve but a further investigation at the hospital was said to show a malfunction of the gall bladder and an operation was suggested but was declined.

A further psionic check-up showed a very definite improvement all round with the precancer reading eliminated and a balance for the first time of the autonomic nervous system. Treatment was now given to deal with the prostate and a Vit E deficiency.

He continued to make good progress, though there was a recurrence of a skin trouble (psoriasis) which he said only bothered him when he was feeling fit! This was duly treated, and when seen a year later he was reported to be in very good health.

Case 31 J. M. W., male, aged 8

This patient had been referred by his doctor for psionic medical diagnosis. He was reported as pale, thin and irritable, with pustules on face and tonsils, and a palpable liver. Despite every care at home he did not seem to make any headway.

Psionic medical analysis revealed the presence of toxins associated with amoebic dysentery (although no gross infection was apparently present when first seen by the reporting physician), with atypical bacillus coli organisms and staphylococcal toxins. There was also a bovine tubercular miasm.

Treatment was commenced, but the patient was then involved in an accident resulting in the fracture of both bones in the right forearm, which failed to respond to treatment. After some eight weeks the doctor wrote 'The X-rays, I am told, show that the bone healing is slow and causing concern to the orthopaedic surgeon and pediatrician. The child is still pale and thin and has some generalized lymph-gland enlargement particularly in neck and axillae. The blood pathology and biochemical tests seem normal. I am sure that this child is not assimilating his food. His mother is particular about giving him the right foods, but even the use of oral comfrey tablets and vitamin and calcium tablets has apparently not helped the fracture to heal. Naturally the parents are worried about the lad. Can you throw any more light on the scene?'

A further analysis was made and appropriate treatment prescribed, as a result of which the patient made an excellent recovery. His mother wrote to the doctor asking him to convey her gratitude. 'Young John,' she wrote, 'is marvellous and in recent weeks is filling out, putting on weight, and is a bundle of energy.'

This case is reported not so much because of the good result but because it illustrates two important characteristics of the psionic medical potential. One is that in diagnosis and prescription, distance is no object and the fact that the patient cannot be seen in person does not preclude successful treatment. In this particular case the patient was as far away as Australia, on the other side of the world.

Second, it is not uncommon to find that in chronic illness in patients who have lived in hot climates, toxins may be present which have been acquired as a result of infection with organisms confined to such climates. The actual infection may have passed unnoticed or may have been treated by orthodox drugs and apparently cured, but psionic medical diagnosis often reveals residual toxins which are not responsive to the drugs and which are causing, often over the years, some chronic complaint which is never associated with the previous infection. This occurs usually because the symptoms bear no relation to those normally associated with the infective stage and the lapse of time, and even the previous medical history, tend to obscure the diagnostic connection.

Case 32 H. G., female, aged 28. Breech presentation correction

This patient, an expectant mother seven months pregnant, sought help for the alleviation of considerable discomfort caused by a very active baby in a breech presentation. At the same time she wished to know if it was possible to correct the abnormal position of the baby so that the likely birth complications could be avoided. The remedy that was chosen—Cicuta Virosa—in homoeopathic potency, has as its main indications a tendency to spasms which bend the head, neck and spine backwards with, probably, turning of the head to one side; also a tendency to convulsions. This appeared to be the position of the foetus in the uterus, which abnormal position had been confirmed by the obstetrician.

The medicine was prescribed twice daily for ten days. On the seventh day the mother reported that the baby changed to normal position in the womb and, later, that it only manifested normal activity thereafter, to her considerable relief. The baby was born in due course and despite the fact that it weighed nine pounds four ounces there were no complications.

It is interesting to note in this case that the mother had previously had treatment, psionically indicated, for removal of miasms and acquired toxins and it is likely that this played a part in the successful outcome. The father had already been cleared of miasms and toxins. This double clearance of both parents before birth was no doubt responsible for the finding that the baby, when checked, had neither miasms nor toxins herself.

Case 33 P. S. H., male, aged 43
First seen in September 1972, the patient reported that he had been suffering from Hodgkin's disease since 1964. Tuberculosis and pneumothorax with onset in 1948 had lasted for six years. Radiations for a neck swelling had been given, the last being in 1970 followed by injections of nitrogen mustard compound. During the treatment half the patient's hair fell out and there were various violent side effects. Immediately prior to seeking psionic medical diagnosis and treatment the doctor had advised a further course of nitrogen mustard to last one year because the swellings had recurred. The patient refused to undergo any further drug treatment. Shingles in 1966, glandular fever in 1956, and pain in prostate gland were also reported during the course of the first consultation. The patient had lived abroad for some years.

The psionic medical analysis revealed the presence of the double tubercular miasm. Treatment with homoeopathic medication was started. Over the next ten weeks three courses were given with excellent effect. The patient then decided to go abroad for the winter, confident that all would be well. In February 1973 a card was received which read: 'Just to tell you that I am feeling very fit and well. Bathing and sun-bathing all day and playing golf and tennis!'

In July he returned to this country and was given a thorough medical examination as a result of which his doctor was completely satisfied and said that no medication was necessary.

Case 34 Nasal haemorrhage

This patient suddenly developed severe nose bleeding which continued for several days despite admission to two hospitals for surgical intervention and packing. Confined to bed, both the loss of blood and the prospect of further continual haemorrhage brought distress to patient and family.

A psionic medical diagnosis was suggested by a friend and this was carried out mainly with a view to getting relief as rapidly as possible, later to be extended in the usual manner to discover miasms and toxins and acquired toxins as underlying causes.

Nasal venous congestion was obviously present but the most commonly used homoeopathic medicines did not appear to be appropriate on psionic indications. Further tests showed that Hirudo—the leech—was indicated and six powders of this medicine in homoeopathic potency were prescribed at twelve-hour intervals. On the following day the patient reported that all bleeding had stopped and he had been free for twenty-four hours. After the powders were finished there was a minor recurrence but this was rapidly controlled and the intention is now to proceed to the removal of the basic miasms which may well have given rise to the situation in which the acute symptoms developed.

The interest in this case lies particularly in the illustration of the homoeopathic principle of 'like cures like'. It is of course well known that the leech has been used for centuries to promote haemorrhage. But it is certainly not so well known that in homoeopathic potency it can be used to stop it; provided it is indicated in the particular case at a particular time.

Case 35 U. D., male, aged 6½. Prophylactic dentistry

This final case is an interesting example of the preventive possibilities of psionic medicine. At the age of 6½ this child shows no evidence of any dental decay whatsoever. His deciduous teeth have erupted and have remained perfect and caries-free. The average child could be expected to exhibit at least half a dozen cavities.

At a few weeks old a psionic analysis was carried out and showed that a double tubercular miasm was present—inherited from both parents. This miasm was removed homoeopathically, thus eliminating the constitutional predisposition to dental caries that is always associated with the tubercular miasm, particularly the bovine variety. Both parents had a poor dental history, which is well known to predispose the offspring to dental disorders, but in this instance the trouble was entirely avoided by early psionic treatment.

Appendix 4

The Formative Forces in Cancer

In a programme on Radio 4 (9 October 1973) four specialists answered questions from the public on the subject of cancer, in the course of which it was said that while a proportion of cases could be cured by modern methods, the basic cause of carcinoma appeared to be some as yet unidentified viruses. This is in entire accord with psionic medical experience in which the basic factors in cancerous conditions are so often found to be inherited miasms or acquired toxins.

Some pertinent comments on the subject were made by Dr Laurence in an article in the *Journal of the Psionic Medical Society* (vol. 1 no. 5) wherein he says:

> When the ovum has been fertilised by the sperm a process of rapid subdivision sets in creating a mass of undifferentiated cells called the morula. Then, by the influence of what Rudolf Steiner calls the Formative Forces (the cosmic formative forces, which we cannot pretend to understand) this mass of cells gradually becomes differentiated into the various parts and organs of the animal or human body. If these forces are interfered with or inhibited things may go wrong. For instance, if the mother develops measles during the first three months of pregnancy quite definite deformations may be produced, such as a hare lip or a hole in the heart. Again if the mother smokes during pregnancy a not uncommon result is a slowing down of both mental and physical development in the child, so that it is always behind other children of the same age, which is a serious handicap. These are immediate and obvious results of a known toxaemia, but a much more common and by no means so obvious a factor is that of inherited toxins or miasms, more usually tubercular but sometimes those of the

venereal diseases. Unfortunately there are no orthodox clinical or laboratory tests for these deep-seated toxins.

Nevertheless, American scientists have discovered (as reported in chapter 5) what appears to be a connection between a wide variety of ills, including some forms of cancer, and what they call 'smouldering viruses' left over from some common infection early in life, such as measles. This bears out the experience of psionic medicine in which there is frequently found a hangover of measles toxins in mental and cancer cases, and indeed, in a very large number of cases of chronic ailments, such as migraine, tinnitus aurium and so on, in which symptomatic treatment can only be palliative until the basic toxins have been eliminated.

So far as the present evidence goes to show, says Laurence, the viruses found in cases of cancer are quite as likely to be produced by the disease as to be the cause of it. This is borne out by the fact that carcinoma is not infectious. He goes on to say:

> To come back to my theme, any factor that can interfere with or inhibit the action of the formative forces can cause the cells in almost any part of the body to revert to the morula stage, that of unrestricted and undifferentiated multiplication, as is found in carcinoma. The fact that cancer cells can spread about the body and cause fresh centres of trouble can be explained by presuming that these migrant cells simply trigger off a reaction which was ready to happen for the same reason as the origin of the primary tumour—the inhibition of the formative forces, which itself may have been started off by trauma or some extra toxin such as tobacco or local irritation as in some occupational cases. We claim that in the majority of cases of cancer the basic cause can be found. Furthermore we have evidence that once the primary tumour has been removed and the basic cause found and eliminated, it is often possible to deal with the secondary deposits and affected glands quite satisfactorily.
>
> I am encouraged in this point of view by no less an authority than Sir MacFarlane Burnet, who in his book *Genes, Dreams and Realities* is not at all optimistic that we will eventually find a cure for every disease—note the word cure—but goes on to say that in western countries at any rate, most ill-health is attributable to physical degeneration processes

which are fundamentally normal to cancer and to mental illness. Professor Burnet argues persuasively that we are programmed by defects in our genetic make-up for diseases which will express themselves if we live long enough. How well this tallies with what we find so often in both inherited and acquired toxaemias, the effects of which may not appear for many years.

The great difficulty, of course, is the fact that these subtle toxins can only be detected by techniques involving extra-sensory perception, but the new climate of medical opinion, which is becoming increasingly concerned with causes as distinct from symptoms, holds the promise of significant advance in the treatment of cancer and other chronic diseases.

Further Reading

BURNET, SIR MACFARLANE (1971). *Genes, Dreams and Realities*, Medical & Technical Publishing Company, London.

HAUSCHKA, RUDOLPH (1966). *The Nature of Substance*, trans. Mary Richards and Marjorie Spock, Vincent Stuart, London.

HEYWOOD, R. (1961). *Beyond the Reach of Sense*, Dutton, New York.

KOESTLER, A. (1972). *The Roots of Coincidence*, Hutchinson, London.

MCDONAGH, J. R. (1966). *Protein—the Basis of all Life*, Heinemann, London.

MERMET, THE ABBÉ (1959). *Principles and Practice of Radiesthesia*, trans. Mark Clement, Vincent Stuart, London.

RAWSON, D. S. (1972). 'A homoeopathtic approach to pollution', *Journal of the American Institute of Homoeopathy*, **65** (2).

REYNER, J. H. (1974). *The Diary of a Modern Alchemist*, Neville Spearman, London.

RHINE, L. E. (1961). *Hidden Channels of the Mind*, Sloane, New York.

RICHARDS, GUYON (1973 reprint). *The Chain of Life*, Health Science Press, London.

ROBERTS, H. A. (1972). *The Principles and Art of Cure by Homoeopathy*, Health Science Press, London.
Observations of a distinguished American homoeopath.

SHERRINGTON, SIR CHARLES (1940). *Man on his Nature*, Cambridge University Press, London.
A wide-ranging expression of a biologist's philosophy originally given as the Gifford Lectures to the University of Edinburgh in 1937–8. Reprinted in a Pelican edition.

TOMLINSON, H. (1953). *The Divination of Disease*, Health Science Press, London.

WATSON, LYALL (1973). *Supernature*, Hodder, London.
A collection of a wide range of authentic paranormal phenomena.

WESTLAKE, A. T. (1961). *The Pattern of Health*, Revised edition, 1973, Shambhala, San Francisco.
Personal experiences with paranormal phenomena, including an account of the secret science of the Kahunas of Polynesia.

WESTLAKE, A. T. (1971). *Life Threatened—Menace and Way Out*, Stuart & Watkins, London.

WHEELER, CHARLES and KENYON, J. D. (1972). *Introduction to the Principles and Practice of Homoeopathy*, Health Science Press, London.

A standard work on the subject.

Reference may also be made to the journals and booklets of the Psionic Medical Society, Hindhead, Surrey, England, notably:

LAURENCE, GEORGE, *Knowing and Affecting by Extra-Sensory Means. The Unitary Conception of Disease in Relation to Radiesthetic Diagnosis.*

SCOTT-ELLIOT, MAJOR-GENERAL J., 'Dowsing in archaeology', *Journal of the Psionic Medical Society*, vol. 1, no. 5.

UPTON, CARL, *The Role of Dowsing in the Development of Psionic Medicine.*

Index

Aberration of protein, 41, 78, 90, 106
Abrams, Albert, 4
Acquired toxins, 71, 81
Allergies, 33, 113, 120
Allopathy, 27, 70, 76, 95
Aluminium toxins, 38, 117, 121
Amino acids, 45, 72
Antibodies, 90
Asthma, 87, 116
Atomic structure, 42

Bach remedies, 68
Bacterial flora, 91, 113
Biochemical imbalance, 75, 95
Biological fall-out, 38, 63, 76
Black holes, 14
Blood spot, 4, 52, 62, 108
British Society of Dowsers, 51, 57, 96
Burnet, Sir MacFarlane, 133

Carcinoma, 34, 132
Causation, 6, 20, 31, 73, 83
Central nervous system, 12
Charts, diagnostic, 58, 67, 103
Chronic conditions, 8, 31, 73
Colloids, 45
Colour, in diagnosis, 69
Compassion, 29
Consciousness, 16 28, 60
Continuous creation, 15, 44
Cosmic influences, 77

Derangements, 6, 32, 41
Diabetes, 35, 74
Diathesis, 36
Diet, 63, 71, 80, 107
Dimensions, meaning of, 19
DNA, 70
Dowsing, 5, 50, 55, 61, 93, 97

Electromagnetic waves, 12
Emanations, 4, 76
Environment, influence of, 78
Epiblast, 108
Eternity, 19, 52
Etheric: body, 17, 31; force fields, 31, 43, 94; realm, 18, 43, 54, 94

Factory husbandry, 64
Faith, 64, 92
Fall-out, 37, 63, 76

Ferris, Dr Elizabeth, 92
Flatlanders, 20
Formative forces, 40, 74, 132
Fourth dimension, 20

Genetic code, 33, 70, 83

Hahnemann, Samuel, 2, 24, 76
Half life, 38
Hangover, 81, 88, 90
Hereditary miasms, 33, 81, 90
Hinton, C. H., 20
Homoeopathic aggravation, 85, 112, 118
Homoeopathy, 2, 24, 70, 95
Horder, Lord, 5
Hypoblast, 108
Hypochondria, 89

Illusion, 13, 43
Imbalance, 38, 69, 75, 95, 96, 106
Immunization, 71
Inference, 18, 68
Integrating influences, 44, 94
Intelligence, 16, 92
Interrogation of samples, 53, 100
Intuition, 15, 50, 92

Knowledge, limitations of, 11, 16
Koestler, Arthur, 11

Lifetime: of elements, 43; of miasms, 38, 63

McDonagh, J. R., 40, 90
Malaria toxins 74, 86
Maya, 13
Measles toxins, 33, 74, 82, 120
Mental illness, 72
'Mentals', 37
Mermet, the Abbé, 5
Mesoblast, 108
Metal poisoning, 39
Miasms, 3, 22, 30, 45, 63, 71; persistence of, 38, 63; in soil, 64
Microdoses, 26
Micro-organisms, 16, 31, 76, 106
Migraine, 73, 86, 111
Mind, nature of, 15, 51, 64
Molecular biology, 70

Negative phase, 85
Nucleic: depletion, 85; energy, 37; fall-out, 37, 76

Octave structure of elements, 42
Odyle, 49
Oral hygiene, 79
Osteopathy, 28

Palliatives, 32
Paranormal senses, 3, 15, 20, 28, 47, 70, 94
Pathogens, 77
Pendulum, 8, 27, 55, 67, 97; misuse of, 62
Perception: extra-sensory, 18, 47, 96; normal range of, 12
Plato's slit, 14, 19
Polarity, in micro-organic life, 77

Polio miasms, 116
Potentizing, 2, 25
Preventive dentistry, 63, 130
Primitive malady, 30, 35
Protein, 41, 45, 70; aberration of 41, 78, 90, 106
Psi functions, 2, 7, 48
Psionic Medical Society, 7, 62, 85
Psora, 31, 36

Quality, change of, 21, 94
Questioning, 56, 67, 100

Radiation, 4, 18, 44, 95
Radiesthesia, 5, 50
Reichenbach, Carl von, 49
Relationships, 52
Remote prescription, 128
Request, 53
Residual toxins, 34, 38, 63, 81, 90
Rhine, J. B., 48
Richards, Guyon, 6
RNA, 70, 89
Roberts, H. A., 36

Salvage dentistry, 81
Saprophytes, 77
Scepticism, 65
Schizophrenia, 89, 123
Scott-Elliot, Major-General J., 57
Senses: limitations of, 13; paranormal, 2, 18, 47, 96
Sensitivity, 47, 70
Sherrington, Sir Charles, 2
Smouldering virus, 34, 133
Space-time continuum, 18
Superspace, 14
Sycosis, 31, 36, 70
Sydenham, Thomas, 31
Symptoms, 9, 71, 96
Syphilitic miasms, 31, 36, 70, 89

Time-body, 52
Tomlinson, H., 38
Toxic fall-out, 37, 63
Toxins, residual, 34, 38, 63, 81, 90
Transformation, 94
Transplant surgery, 72
Tubercular miasms, 33, 73, 82, 87, 112

Unitary theory of disease, 40, 73, 106
Unmanifest realm, 9, 11, 20, 94

Vaccinosis toxins, 82, 88
Vibrations, 12, 18
Vis Medicatrix Naturae, 22, 25, 85, 95
Vis occulta, 49
Vital energy, 6, 11, 22, 26, 77, 94
Vitality, 32, 39, 71
Vitamin deficiency, 82, 113

Water divining, 5, 50, 101
Watson, Lyall, 93
Westlake, A. T., 8, 33, 49
Wheeler, John A., 14
Witnesses, 58, 62, 68